POWERFUL COACHING: COACHING TOOLS TO REACH YOUR GREATEST POTENTIAL

MAX CHAHUA

Copyright © 2021 Max Chahua

All rights reserved.

ISBN: 9798523494185

DEDICATION

To my parents, for their support.

CONTENT

INTRODUCTION 1

SECTION I- TYPES OF COACHING 3

SECTION II –CONCEPTS Y BASIC DEFINITIONS IN COACHING 6

1 – BARRIERS AND LIMITING BELIEFS 7

2 – LEARNING ZONES 16

3 - ACTUAL STATE, DESIRED STATE AND THE GAP 25

4 - THE LINGUISTIC ACTS 29

5 - TYPES OF STATEMENTS 38

6 - REASONS WHY WE LOSE OPPORTUNITIES TO LEARN 41

7 JUGDGEMENTS 45

8 BREAK OR BREAKDOWN 49

9 THE COMPLAINT 53

10 WORDS 55

11 - ELEMENTS THAT DEFINE A PERSON 57

12 - EMOTIONS THAT BLOCK LEARNING 58

13 - LEARNING MODALITIES 62

14 - LEARNING STYLES 67

15 - OBSERVER TRANSFORMATION 70

16 - MENTAL MODELS 72

17- MOODS 79

18 - CONVERSATIONS 82

19 - THE LANGUAGE 86

20 - MOTIVATION 88

21 - HOW TO END BAD HABITS 95

22 - USE OF THE 3 DOMAINS 105

23 - COACHING AS AN ALARM CLOCK 110

24 - MASTERY WHEN ASKING	111
SECTION III- COACHING TOOLS	112
TOOL #1 – GROW MODEL	113
TOOL #2 – SMART GOALS	118
TOOL #3 - ALTERNATIVE FUTURES	124
TOOL #4 – WHEEL OF LIFE	131
TOOL #5 - PROCESS GOALS VS RESULT GOALS	135
TOOL #6 - THE LEFT COLUMN	139
TOOL #7 - THE CIRCLE OF EXCELLENCE	144
TOOL #8 – PPEAR MODEL	147
TOOL #9 - ANCHOR TECHNIQUE	153
TOOL #10 - TECHNIQUES OF THE 15 OPTIONS	156
FINAL NOTES	158
ABOUT THE AUTHOR	160
FINAL EXERCISE	161

ACKNOWLEDGMENTS

My deep gratitude to all those people who positively influenced my life.

INTRODUCTION

I started in coaching doing a coaching diploma, there, I learned different types of coaching, such as life coaching, executive coaching, ontological coaching, coaching with NLP, systemic coaching and some sports coaching.

In this diploma, I learned a lot about coaching and the tools of each type of coaching.

Based on this diploma, my interest in coaching increased and I developed as an Ontological coach, currently I am certified as an Ontological Coach.

Coaching is a powerful tool and has its origins in Socrates' maieutics, which is a technique that he applied 2,500 years ago.

The maieutics was used by Socrates for teaching, it consisted of asking questions so that the student discovers in himself the answers to his questions.

Through this technique Socrates made people discover solutions and concepts that were hidden within the mind of each student.

In coaching, maieutics is applied by creating a questionnaire which guides the inner wisdom of the person.

The maieutics begins with asking simple questions and little by little go exploring in more depth within the reasoning of the interviewee.

Uncomfortable questions are also asked that force us to think and challenge us, take us out of our comfort zone, go through anger, frustration, paradoxes that lead the interviewee or the coachee to be honest with themselves.

Coaching does not seek to heal sick people, coaching is not psychology, what coaching seeks is to get the maximum potential of people.

Coaching is a way to achieve your best version of yourself.

Coaching can cover various areas such as personal, business, professional, sports, according to the requirement of the person.

Coaching is not counseling.

Coaching develops differently for each person as each person has different needs and goals.

What coaching seeks is to take you from a situation from a situation that is unsatisfactory (Point A) to a point B which is the ideal or dreamed situation and through questions, we can visualize the ways to reach that desired point.

There are several coaching tools, in this book some of them will be shown, however, coaching is not only the tools, coaching covers various areas, the tools are a part of coaching, but also ethics, the understanding of language, and other concepts are part of coaching.

What I'm looking for with this book is that you can empower yourself by making use of these powerful coaching tools.

Section I explains in detail the existing types of Coaching.

In Section II, basic concepts of coaching process are defined.

Section III shows coaching tools that belong to different types of Coaching.

You can use these techniques on yourself to start, if you are a coach, you can apply these tools with your coachees (clients).

SECTION I- TYPES OF COACHING

There are several types of coaching.

People seek to improve their performance, and improve their capabilities, because of this, there are different types of coaching.

Depending on the objectives to be achieved and the preferences of a person there are different coaching alternatives.

Depending on the type of method used, we have:

-Ontological Coaching- It is oriented to the optimal use of language, linguistic processes and tools. It relies on language, emotions, and conversations to generate change.

Use language to generate change.

It speaks of the generative language, through which a new world and a reality can be generated.

It uses concepts such as distinctions, breaks, judgments, and others, to treat coaching from the field of language.

Referents in this area we have Rafael Echevarria (Ontology of Language), Humberto Maturana, Leonardo Wolk, among others.

I am formed as an Ontological coach, so many concepts that we will deal with, as well as tools will come from this type of coaching.

-Systemic Coaching - The person is seen as part of a system, and as such has a certain behavior. The subject, being part of a system, has limited the changes that he can make. The system or environment can limit or extend the changes that a person can make.

Sometimes when looking to make changes through other types of coaching, no changes are generated or very few are generated (such as Ontological Coaching or Life Coaching).

Systemic coaching makes an evaluation about this, and details that this could be due to the "system" that surrounds it.

In other words, sometimes the system can limit the development or change of a person, because it is delimited by it.

-Coercive Coaching - This type of coaching uses high-impact techniques, such as walking on hot coals, among others.

-Coaching with Emotional Intelligence - Based on Goleman's contributions on emotional intelligence. It seeks to achieve improvements in the person through the use and proper management of emotional intelligence.

-NLP Coaching (Neuro Linguistic Programming) - This type of coaching combines coaching with Neuro Linguistic programming. Analyzing how the person interprets and faces reality.

Programming - All behavior derives from a certain mental "program".

Neuro- Its base is in the brain.

Linguistics- Language is what distinguishes it from other living things.

According to NLP, we move through life, responding to our own personal model of the world.

In other words, each person has a certain "programming" that makes them act in a certain way. These "programs" can benefit or harm us.

Through NLP one can be aware of their own mental programs, and allows us to free ourselves from those programming that harm us.

If you are aware of your internal programming, and that it hurts you, you can shape it and change it to your advantage.

Richard Bandler and Grinder are important references in this area.

-Cognitive Coaching - This type of coaching allows the effective transmission of knowledge in a coaching process. It takes into account cognitive functions, memory, learning and thinking.

Types of coaching according to the purpose we have:

-Life Coaching - Provides support to people seeking a significant change in their lives. You work on life projects, personal mission, personal goals, etc. Pursuing personal well-being.

-Coaching for the development of skills - This type of coaching program focuses on achieving specific skills, which are linked to the organization.

-Organizational Coaching (business and executive) - They are linked to the professional field, and are developed within an organizational context.

-Executive Coaching - Focused on improving the performance of managers and seeking improvements in workers and in the company

-Business Coaching- It is aimed at organizations or companies in general. They deal with topics such as time management, productivity, relationship with workers, etc.

-Sports Coaching - It works on the development and potential of the athlete, seeking to improve his performance.

SECTION II –CONCEPTS Y BASIC DEFINITIONS IN COACHING

In this section We will deal with important topics in order to understand coaching and its tools.

We will deal with topics such as: declarations, affirmations, judgments, breaks, mental models, learning styles, among others.

These concepts are important to understand the coaching process as well as to understand its tools.

1 – BARRIERS AND LIMITING BELIEFS

At times we want to do something, but many times we do not feel capable of achieving it, this could be because we have limiting beliefs.

These limiting beliefs often prevent us from growing.

These limiting beliefs are usually illusions that we build in our heads and that place limits on our growth.

The story of the elephant and the stake is famous.

Let me tell you briefly:

The story goes that there was a baby elephant, which ran, ran and walked along the wide field, but the owner of it, to prevent it from getting lost and moving away, tied the elephant to a small stake.

Imagine the hours that the little elephant tried to get away from that stake and thus, day after day it kept trying, as time went by, the elephant gave up on getting out of the stake, believing that it could "never" get out of the stake.

Many years later, when this elephant was an adult (and capable of felling trees, due to his enormous weight and enormous strength), when his master tied him to the stake, the elephant no longer insisted on getting out of the stake.

The elephant did not believe it possible to get away from the stake even though he was already an adult elephant and possessed colossal strength.

If the elephant wanted to, it could knock down trees, but in the elephant's mind it couldn't get out of the stake!

The idea that it was impossible to get out of this stake had been internalized within this elephant.

Although at the beginning getting out of the stake was unlikely for the little elephant in this story, later on as it gained more mass and strength it was possible to get out of the stake.

How many of us are clinging to old ideas, believing that we cannot achieve or achieve something? But now many years later, with new tools and skills, perhaps we are able now to get rid of some of our mental "stakes".

Phrases like:

"When I achieve this ... (whatever it is) I will succeed"

"When I have this or that tool, I can be successful"

"When I have money, I will be able to undertake"

While these phrases have some truth, there are many things we can do even if we have little money, even if we do not have certain tools.

These types of phrases limit us.

In some cases, we could expect certain things to have certain advantages and operate, which would be advantageous.

For example, you could wait for a certain amount of money to start a business, or master a certain skill to start something you want.

The danger, however, is that these things that we hope for **may be excuses** for not doing something we want to do, and inside we are really afraid of doing it, and that we are hiding behind these apparent logical reasons.

The best way to see if this was an excuse or not, is to do what you say after reaching what you said you were missing, for example, if you said that you needed to acquire a certain skill to do what you said, then the most logical thing is to do it, once you have acquired the skill you mentioned, otherwise it was an excuse.

Let me tell you a couple of short personal stories that have to do with the story of the elephant and the stake in my personal life.

FIRST STORY

"When I have money, I will start my business"

It turns out that I had always had the desire to undertake, for which I considered that I needed a certain amount of money to start.

Since I did not have that amount of money, I had the perfect excuse not to start my business.

So, some years passed, I dedicated myself to working in a company, and I began to accumulate and save money.

There came a time when I had the amount of money, I needed to start that business and maybe a little more.

So why didn't I start with my business?

Money was no longer an excuse.

But then other types of excuses began to appear, now it was no longer the money, but now it was "I have no time."

Possibly the truth was that I was "scared to death."

I was dying of fear that what I wanted to achieve so much (starting a business and being successful in it) might not be successful, before which I froze with fear.

These internal fears were translated into logical explanations through apparently logical phrases such as "I have no money", then it was "I am not afraid", but they hid the truth.

The truth was, I was afraid of failure.

Fear that what he wanted so badly to achieve would end in failure, and that I would lose money.

The result?

The result was that my fear was fulfilled.

It turns out that I did not undertake, and anyway I lost a lot of money and that everything was a fiasco.

The lesson?

After having lost a lot of money and a lot of time.

I realized and admitted the truth, that I was afraid, that I was full of excuses, and that if I ran out of excuses (as in the case of "I have no money or I have no time"), I would make new excuses.

This made me think deeply.

And it made me do away with this limiting belief that "it takes a lot of money to start a business."

Having money to start a business can be important, but this does not have to be a limitation.

From this experience, I no longer allowed the lack of money to be an excuse to undertake.

Since there are many investments that can be made with little capital, it is true that there are ventures that do need a lot of money to start.

But because I did not want the limiting belief that "you have to have a lot of money to start", I started to start in businesses that needed little capital.

SECOND STORY

This story shows how powerful the mind can be.

When I was young there was a game that I liked to play, there were 2 ways to play it, the first with a keyboard and the other with a game controller (used in play station).

It turns out that I saw that the most expert played with a controller, while I always played with a keyboard, and according to my logic, therefore, I did not win many games.

I said: "They win because they have a game controller, and I don't win much because I use the keyboard."

It turns out that one day I bought a controller and started playing with it, the result?

It turned out that I was much worse with the controller, and with it, my excuse and limiting belief died.

What happened next?

That I used the keyboard again, but this time I was winning many more games, because this limiting barrier died.

When this happened to me, I started to think about:

How many things do we think we think we need to be better, but if we would have them, maybe there wouldn't be much difference?

Is the mind so powerful that when I realized that this excuse was false, now I won more easily?

How many other excuses do I have in other areas of life that could be limiting me?

I started to think of many phrases that people usually say such as:

"If I had more time"

"If I had had the proper education"

"If I had taken this or that course"

"If I had studied this or that thing"

"if I had money"

"If I were successful"

"If my partner will help me"

"If I would be younger"

"If it would be a little older"

"If I had that tool that the competition has"

"If I would have the means that my greatest rival has"

…

"If I had a game controller" in my case

And what if we would have what we say we lack, would we really do it, would we really be successful?

As I repeat, it could be that we need some tools to improve our productivity, or we need a certain amount of money to undertake, for example, these could be valid reasons.

However, let us be very careful that these deficiencies, instead of valid reasons, are disguised excuses, to really know if it is one or the other, we have to be honest with ourselves and analyze in detail if it is one or the other.

EXERCISE

Identify some limiting barriers you had in the past

_____
_____
_____
_____

_____

Identify limiting barriers that you currently have and identify if they are really impediments and logical reasons, or are they excuses disguised as logical reasons?

_____
_____
_____
_____

_____

How to overcome the limiting barriers?

Many times, we believe that we do not deserve what we want, this could be due to childhood experiences.

Many times, we want to make changes in our life, but we do not make them because of some thoughts that prevent us from trying.

Our limiting beliefs are influenced by our experiences in our environment, childhood experiences, social experiences, and our own personality.

Some things you can do to overcome your limiting barriers are to work your mind and spirit, meditate, work on yourself, and work on your personal growth.

We can't change the past, but we can change the way we view our past, we can also change our present, and by changing our present we can shape our future.

The best way to overcome our limiting barriers is by identifying which are those limiting beliefs, which could be holding us back, and modifying them.

Once these limiting beliefs have been identified, we move on to what is called "killing sacred cows" and then making new phrases.

Some sacred cows that I killed as I mentioned were:

SACRED COW 1

- "I need a lot of money to start a business"

Now in my mind is:

"Although it is important to have money to be able to start a business, this is not necessarily a limitation, and in the worst-case scenario I can start a business with little investment"

SACRED COW 2

-In order to achieve these results, I need "x" tool

Now in my mind is:

"Although that tool is important and I do not have it yet, there are other things I can do to achieve good results, until I get that tool"

EXERCISE

Identify your limiting beliefs, kill your sacred cows, and reformulate them

Limiting belief 1

_____

_____

Reformulate

_____

_____

Limiting belief 2

_____

_____

Reformulate

_____

_____

Limiting belief 3

_____

_____

Reformulate

_____

_____

2 – LEARNING ZONES

Learning is growing. Learning has 3 zones. The first is the comfort

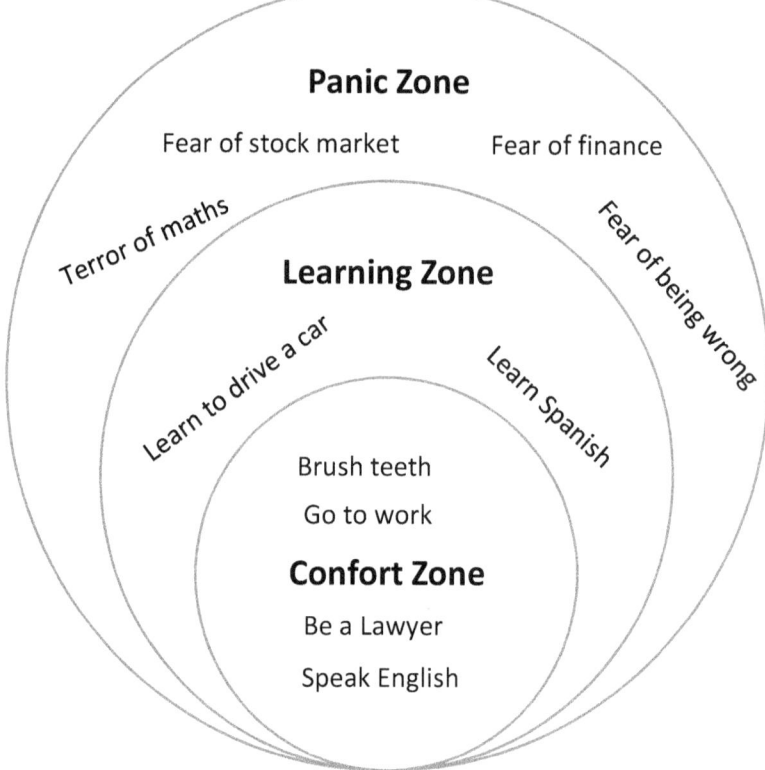

zone, the second is the learning zone or expansion zone, and last we have the fear zone or panic zone, which induces us to return to the first zone.

Example of a person's learning zones.

In this person's comfort zone, is what he always does and is already a habit, such as brushing his teeth, going to work, speaking his native language, practicing his legal profession.

In his expansion zone, things that he is currently doing to expand his expansion zone, in this case, the person is learning to drive and is learning an additional language.

Finally, in his fear zone, are the fears that afflict him, and his prejudices on certain issues, this person is afraid of the stock market, for example, which freezes him, and slows him down. He is also afraid of finances and money management.

This person grew up with the idea that he isn't good for mathematics, and he is also afraid of being wrong because at school he was made fun of, every time he answered wrong.

THE COMFORT ZONE

It is that area where we feel comfortable, where we already have the knowledge acquired where we operate on automatic pilot, this comfort zone is expanding over the years.

For example, when you don't know how to drive, or you can't swim, this is out of your comfort zone, but once you master them, they become part of your comfort zone and you can even do it on autopilot.

The way to expand the comfort zone is through the expansion zone or learning zone, once we are in our comfort zone it is easy for us to do these types of activities, if we want to expand our knowledge and skills, we have to expand our comfort zone, we achieve this through the expansion or learning zone.

Is it wrong to have a comfort zone?

No, since this comfort zone helps us save energy when we drive, for example, we do it many times without realizing it, when we get up and do our activities, many of them forget that we did them.

For example, when we brush sometimes, we don't even remember that we have done it, we just did it automatically as part of our routine.

Having activities as habits helps us save a lot of energy and allows us to live in a faster, simpler and more effective way.

The knowledge acquired in any area allows us to work with greater effectiveness and productivity, the bad thing in this case would be not to expand our comfort zone and stay there in that known world and not expand it.

Our comfort zone widens over time and with age, for example, when we were babies, walking was a challenge for us, and it was part of our expansion zone, once we were able to walk well, it was already part of our comfort zone., expanding this zone.

EXPANSION/LEARNING ZONE

Learning occurs in this area, this area is unlimited since science is unlimited, we have sciences to discover and very broad sciences, such as physics, chemistry, astronomy, medicine, law, accounting, finance, psychology, and so on.

In this area, more energy is expended, because learning consumes more energy.

Learning is spent 3 to 4 times more energy than we need when we are in our comfort zone.

In order to learn we have to leave our comfort zone, this exit from the comfort zone also requires a **declaration of ignorance** (there is something I do not know), because if one believes that he knows everything, there is nothing to learn, then there is no expansion zone.

Also in this area, virtues are required, such as: **constancy and perseverance, since learning is a process.**

By learning we are expanding our capacity for action, and once we have learned or internalized much of the learning, it will become part of the comfort zone.

Admitting that one does not know something, part of humility, humility is an important virtue, hence the biblical phrase that says: "the meek will inherit the earth" (Matthew 5: 5-8)

Understanding the humble as meek, that is, those people who never stop learning.

Meekness means: softness and gentleness in condition or treatment, and **is free from arrogance or presumption**.

The biblical phrase does not say the strong, it does not say the intelligent, it does not say the fast, it says the meek will inherit the earth.

This is important to take into account, since we must constantly be updated and constantly expand our knowledge, that is, as far as possible, expand our learning zone or expansion zone.

Today, more important than knowing the correct answers, is having the ability to learn quickly and the ability to unlearn, because many ideas that previously worked today stopped working.

We have to unlearn to learn new things.

For example, 20 or 30 years ago owning your own premises, such as an office or a store, gave presence and power to a large company.

Companies like Walmart were very powerful, however, today, in the information age, having a company with a large location makes it have very high costs and does not allow it to compete against those companies that do not have these locations and that many they operate from their homes and work online through the internet.

For its part, arrogance, which is the opposite, does not allow one to learn, since it is a false belief that we believe that we know everything and we close ourselves in knowledge, we stop learning, limiting or completely closing our learning zone.

FEAR ZONE

You cannot learn in this area, since **where there is fear there is no learning.**

When we are afraid, we want to be safe, if we constantly see that our environment humiliates or punishes those who make mistakes.

What are we going to want?

Well, we will not want to make mistakes, we will not want to learn, we will want to go unnoticed, hide our ignorance, but this will limit us since instead of learning we will have very important areas which will not be covered by knowledge and our comfort zone will be very limited.

We will externalize it with behaviors such as arrogance and hypocrisy, which are nothing more than masks that hide our ignorance and our fear.

How then to respond to the bad conditioning that punishes learning, that punishes error?

Well, understand through adequate knowledge that learning is not bad, that making mistakes is not bad and generating a context of personal trust and respect where one has confidence in oneself, and is not afraid of making mistakes and in a context where we can develop effectively by making mistakes without being judged.

That is the attitude that a person must have in order to expand its comfort zone and its learning zone, since the only way to learn is by making mistakes.

If children were afraid of making a mistake, they would never learn to walk, since they do it by falling, that is why it is important to learn and not be afraid of making a mistake, since if we are afraid of making a mistake, we will not advance and it will be very limited to our area of comfort and our learning zone.

What avoids or minimizes fear is knowledge and education.

Through education and experience, fears are put aside. For one to be able to educate oneself, one has to put aside prejudices on certain subjects, and also put aside personal prejudices, such as "I am not good for mathematics", "I am not good at letters".

EXERCISE

Recreate your personal learning zones.

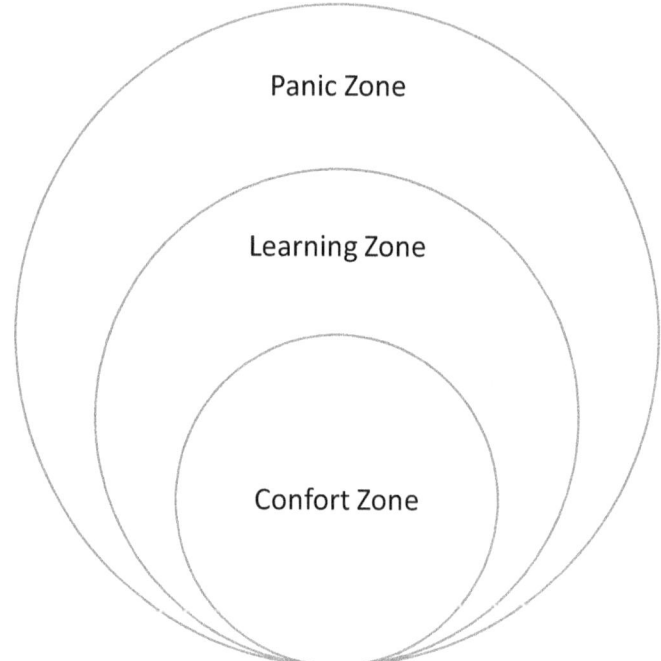

Indicate in each area which activities and topics are part of your Comfort Zone. Which are part of your learning zone and which are your Fear Zone (panic).

Fill each area with the activities you do.

What activities are currently part of your comfort zone?

_____

_____

_____

What activities are currently part of your learning zone?

_____

_____

_____

What activities are part of your fear zone?

_____

_____

_____

_____

What activities a few years ago were part of your panic or learning zone but now form your comfort zone? What do you think this change of area was due to?

_____

_____

_____

_____

What activities would you like to stop being part of your fear zone and become part of your learning zone?

_____

_____

_____

_____

Because knowledge is unlimited there are many topics and areas that we do not know or know little about.

However, you can choose which of these topics and activities that are part of your fear zone are limiting you (due to prejudices that you might have, for example), in order to bring them into your learning zone and finally learn about those topics that can be relevant in your life.

Finally, after learning those topics and areas for a while, at some point they will become part of your comfort zone, helping to expand your comfort zone.

3 - ACTUAL STATE, DESIRED STATE AND THE GAP

The actual or present state is the state you are currently in.

The desired state is the state you would like to be in.

The distance that separates you between your current state and the ideal state is what is called in gap coaching.

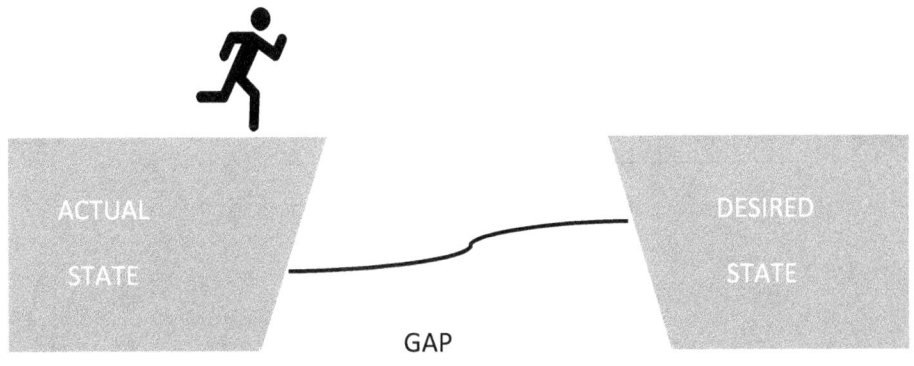

In order to reach the desired state, we have to create a "bridge" to move from the real state to the desired state.

This "bridge" will be everything necessary to reach the desired state, such as knowledge, the necessary tools, work, effort and learning.

We all have beliefs about ourselves, beliefs can empower or limit us.

Coaching is a process of self-discovery.

EXERCISE OF SELF-DISCOVERY AND MOOD

-Throughout the day describe your state of mind.

_____
_____

-Throughout the day listen and write down some of the words and thoughts you have about yourself.

_____
_____

-Evaluate your beliefs and perceptions you have about yourself.

_____
_____

-Write some of the thoughts you have had in those days about yourself.

_____
_____

-Write a reflection of all the aforementioned

_____

_____

-Check if this description of yourself is there, it is the perception that you would like to have under a desired state.

_____

_____

In some cases, we want a new ideal state, because times change.

With globalization many things have changed, perhaps what we knew today is no longer useful to us now.

Maybe it served us in the past, but we realize that it no longer serves us or will no longer serve us in the future, that is why we want to learn new things and be updated.

We are aware that the things we did before that were successful for us today are no longer as effective, before which we need to learn and train in new areas.

We must learn to live under these changes since in life, due to our own personal, professional and financial growth of each person, each time they will present us with greater challenges.

For example, if you are an employee who later becomes a manager, you will have new responsibilities and you will need to have new tools to be able to face that new position.

And so, in various areas of life we will have more and more responsibilities, before which we will need to make changes.

It can also happen that many of the objectives that we have proposed have not been achieved in the way we want, under this scenario we must evaluate what things we have done and what things we can improve to achieve the result we want.

It is important that all our potential is directed towards a goal and that we have certainty of the goals that we want to achieve and we have to be congruent (our goals must not contradict each other).

Our goals must be directed towards an objective so that in this way we can concentrate all our forces on this goal.

Many of our habits tend to imprison us and prevent us from doing the things we really want, when these bad habits are excessive and cannot be controlled, we reach the degree of addiction that can destroy us.

To achieve and achieve the things we want, many of our recurring activities we do, we have to turn them into habits.

4 - THE LINGUISTIC ACTS

We have 2 types of languages, a language that is merely descriptive (passive nature of language), that is, it describes what it sees around it.

Like, for example: "the wall is green", "the earth is brown".

But we also have a generative language, that is to say that through language we can create new realities.

Like, for example: "I'm going to be a doctor", "I'm going to pass this subject."

By making these kinds of statements, I am creating a new reality, and from this statement, I am creating a new world or reality. (to the extent that I comply)

From this perspective we can say that language is action. And that language also has an active nature. (J.L. Austin mentions the performing nature of language.)

Among the linguistic acts we have affirmations, statements, requests.

AFFIRMATIONS AND DECLARATIONS

Rafael Echevarria mentions the following in his book Ontology of Language:

"Does the word fit the world, or does the world fit the word? ...

If the word fits the world and therefore the world leads the word, we are talking about AFFIRMATIONS. If, on the contrary, the word modifies the world, and therefore the world adapts to the word, we are talking about DECLARATIONS. "

AFFIRMATIONS

Statements serve to describe what we see.

For example, if there is a table and I say the word "table" I am describing it, it is to name what we see and express what we observe.

The statements can be true or false according to the evidence accepted by others, when something is accepted by several people given their culture, customs, a social convention is generated, which makes these statements true for this group.

Affirmations also have to do with facts, concrete experiences that are shared by a group of people.

Affirmations correspond to the type of linguistic act that we normally call **descriptions.**

Statements look like descriptions, but they are nonetheless propositions about our observations.

DECLARATIONS

It is the most powerful form of language, it shows the active nature of language, through declarations language is generative and allows things to happen.

Declarative words are prior to reality and **can transform the world,** think about how many things have changed in your personal life from a couple of words spoken. Statements like:

"I'm going to study medicine"

"I'm going to pass my exam"

"I'm going to study Spanish", statements of this type can create new realities, by making statements we are making decisions, we give the possibility of creating new contexts and the possibility of building a new future.

Statements are classified as valid or invalid according to the conferred authority of the speaker.

For example.

Saying "I am going to get to Mars" by a person without the capacity or the resources, because it is simply an invalid statement, on the other hand, if a developed country like the US does it and says "that it is going to get to Mars", then that statement may be valid.

So, the statement depends a lot on the authority of the person who says it, when you declare what you want to be, how you want to be in the future, what you are going to study, what you intend to do, where you plan to work, mark a before and after those words.

An important declaration was the declaration of independence of Peru by Simón Bolívar:

"Peru is from this moment free and independent by the general will of the peoples and for the justice of their cause that God defends. Long live the homeland! Long live freedom! Live the independence!"

From this phrase, and the power of language created a new reality, the world adapted to the words of Simón Bolívar, and from that day on, Peru was independent.

Understanding this, we can denote how powerful words are, and their ability to generate new realities.

We can use it to our advantage by making powerful statements that benefit us and acting consistently on what is said.

Or, on the contrary, we could be making statements that could harm us without realizing it, taking away our power.

If I say, for example:

"I am not good for mathematics"

Is it a declaration or an affirmation? Am I describing reality, or are my words creating my reality? Something to question right?

That is why it is much important to take care of our words.

Declarations can give one power, what is declared has to be consistent with the action, since, once a statement is made, the commitment to be fulfilled is established to be valid, it is important to emphasize the degree of trust that this person has, by giving these statements.

If the person is an honest person with a high reputation and highly respected, it is most likely that he will comply with what he says, if on the contrary, the person is considered a charlatan and who speaks for the sake of talking, then the statement would not have much weight since We know that this person most likely does not comply with what he says, that is the importance of a person's reputation and his words.

There is a phrase of Napoleon that says: "The last to promise is the most faithful to fulfill"

Those people who do what they said have a great reputation for which they are respected and are entrusted with many things.

When we make declarations, we don't talk about the world, we create a new world for ourselves. The word generates a different reality. After what was said has been said, the world is no longer the same as before.

This was transformed by the power of the word.

Some of the declarations that shaped the world are the Declaration of Independence of the United States, the declaration of Winston Churchill to resist fiercely in World War II, the declaration of the rights of man and of the citizen of 1789 in France, etc.

EXERCISE

MENTION SOME STATEMENTS YOU MENTIONED IN YOUR LIFE THAT SHAPED YOUR REALITY

_____

_____

_____

_____

MENTION SOME STATEMENTS MADE BY FAMOUS CHARACTERS WHO SHAPED THE WORLD AND CREATED NEW REALITIES

_____

_____

IMPORTANCE OF DECLARATIONS

As we mentioned, declarations make the world conform to the word.

The declarations are of importance since they give us a direction, they establish a vision.

The declarations are also fulfilled depending on the person who says them, if this person is upright and committed to what he says, his statement has great power.

If, on the other hand, we consider that the person is a charlatan or a liar, his statement could be considered invalid

An example that I like a lot, of the declarations, and of how the world adapts to the word, we have for example

The Declaration of John F. Kennedy to go to the moon.

"We choose to go to the Moon, we choose to go to the Moon in this decade and do those other things, not because it is easy but because it is difficult. Because this goal will serve to organize and test the best of our energies and abilities. Because this challenge is one that we are willing to take on. A challenge that we are not willing to postpone ... and one that we intend to win."

The world adapted to his words, and in that decade, man reached the moon in 1969, of that same decade.

As we can see, people can make statements, companies can make statements and governments can make statements, these statements can shape their world.

As we can see, the statements direct our energy and thought towards concrete objectives.

DECLARATIONS OF PEOPLE

People make declarations, in the new year, all before it touches midnight, we write down our objectives on a paper.

For example:

- ☐ Learn a language
- ☐ Travel to Machu Picchu
- ☐ Do an emotional intelligence seminar
- ☐ Increase my income by "x"

And objectives like that, their fulfillment will depend on the commitment and integrity that the person possesses.

DECLARATIONS OF BUSINESS

Companies also make declarations.

Once the year is over, companies look at their results and show them to their workers, they verify if they fulfilled the commitments they made at the beginning of the year.

They then make declarations for the new year, such as:

- ☐ Grow sales by 10%
- ☐ Reduce our costs by 3%
- ☐ Increase profitability by 5%.
- ☐ Grow 5%, the number of clients.

While these are objectives, they are also declarations, as once written, these statements have the power to make the world conform to the words written and spoken.

One of the most relevant statements in these years was the one made by Elon Musk, of reaching Mars by 2025, and sending a million people to Mars by 2050.

GOVERNMENT DECLARATIONS

Governments also make declarations, as we saw in the case of Kennedy and the United States government.

More examples of government statements are:

☐ Reduce the fiscal deficit by 4%

☐ Increase gold reserves by 3%

☐ Increase the wealth of the country, and reduce social inequality

☐ Reduce poverty by 10%

☐ Increase GDP by 5%, during the next 10 years.

☐ Achieve social prosperity, through the growth of GDP in "x" %, and the increase of economic reserves

As we can see, the declarations are made with the aim of shaping our world, and making the world conform to the word, making use of the active power of language.

The declarations allow us to have a north and focus our attention.

Unlike the passive nature of language that merely describes the world (affirmations).

As we could also see, declarations have the power to shape the world, only if the person who says it has the integrity and commitment to achieve what they say.

EXERCISE

Now that we know the active power of language through statements and its importance, let's do the following exercise

MAKE POWERFUL STATEMENTS AIMING THAT THE WORLD COMES TO YOUR WORDS AND ESTABLISHES THE DEGREE OF COMMITMENT AND INTEGRITY OF YOUR STATEMENTS

_____
_____
_____
_____
_____
_____
_____
_____

5 - TYPES OF STATEMENTS

There are types of statements such as the following:

-Declaration of No
-Declaration of Yes
-Declaration of Ignorance
-Declaration of Gratitude
-Declaration of Forgiveness
-Declaration of Love

We will explain some of these declarations

Declaration of Ignorance

The declaration of ignorance is the act of declaring "I do not know", there are many people who avoid making this declaration since they feel when saying it, diminished, that they exhibit their weaknesses.

This difficulty in expressing their ignorance is linked to certain circumstances or contexts, there are those who are afraid to declare this at work, because it assumes that the important thing about him is to show everything he knows, that is why they hired us.

A father is inhibited from saying that because of his ignorance in front of his children since he does not want to look bad before them, who respect him.

By not making this statement we are compromising our ability to learn, in this way we are prolonging our ignorance, this also has an effect on our system and environment, since the participants are also afraid to declare their ignorance and declare that there is something they do not know.

Ultimately, this social system ends up restricting their ability to learn.

Because we also learn by imitation, it has a modeling effect on children and young people who deny this declaration of ignorance and finally the restrictive effects multiply towards the whole society.

If, on the contrary, in society it is admitted that something is not known and ignorance is admitted, it is possible to learn and reinforce its capacity for learning as a society and reinforce this system.

What are the fears that do as individuals not recognize what they do not know?

Many of these fears in many cases are often unfounded.

There is a phrase that says "we are all ignorant, we just ignore different things"

In reality, we know very little about what we do not know, hence we need to be humble in order to learn and learn to say "I don't know."

Another reason why you do not want to use that declaration of ignorance, is because due to age, many times we are ashamed to see that people younger than us know certain skills and out of shame we deny that we do not know something, but as I repeat this only extends our ignorance.

As the phrase goes: "the humble / meek will inherit the earth".

It does not say the arrogant, it does not say the old, it does not say the intelligent, it says the meek.

That is the importance of the declaration of ignorance, the fear of not recognizing our ignorance simply leads us to prolong it, it is a way of hiding what we do not know.

If we want to move forward, we need to overcome this ignorance, and it is achieved through the declaration of ignorance.

The declaration of ignorance is the beginning to learn.

For autonomous learning this is an irreplaceable tool.

6 - REASONS WHY WE LOSE OPPORTUNITIES TO LEARN

Many times, the perceptions we have of ourselves can block our learning.

For example: the statement "I don't like numbers" blocks us in our learning of mathematics.

Another example is "I chose a law career because I don't like numbers"

And phrases of this type that only extend our ignorance and do not allow us to advance.

Another well-known phrase is "I already know that"

Just because you've read something about a topic in a book doesn't mean you actually know it, since you can't learn to swim from a book.

To learn you need to do things.

"The real learning is action, everything else is information." Einstein

You can only say that you know when you do something.

You can only say that you know how to swim, when you swim.

If you have read a book about swimming, you cannot say that you know how to swim.

What you can say is that you have the information about what swimming is.

Learning is action.

How much money and how many opportunities have been lost because we thought we knew something, but it turned out that we didn't really know it!

One of the main advantages that children have over adults is precisely that children do not have assumptions to defend, they do not have preconceptions, they do not have so much mental garbage, they do not have so many prejudices.

Children have a predisposition to learn and have no preconceptions.

Children live in the world of wonder. Here also resides his innocence.

Jesus said: "to get to the world of heaven you have to be a child since the world of heaven belongs to them."

Another important aspect to note is that children tend to be more gullible.

Chris Gardner in his book "Start Where You Are" mentions the following:

"… I didn't know that you couldn't launch an institutional investment company in Chicago, of all places, with just ten thousand dollars of capital, a phone and a stack of business cards,

in a bubble economy that, without I knew was about to explode ...
"

If you educate a child and tell him that he can be successful at any age at any time, well he will believe it, if, on the contrary, you tell him that he does not deserve success and that he is not good, he will believe it too.

Let's understand the importance of this: how many times do we reinforce negative thoughts in our children?

If we do not have negative preconceptions that limit us, we can achieve success much faster, since we are not afraid.

To be successful you have to act as if you are always successful in the things you do.

To be successful in entrepreneurship, we have to think as if all of our businesses were successful.

An adult is more defensive, regarding his ideas and beliefs.

Every time we have an opportunity for improvement or a problem in our life, we are presented with a great learning opportunity.

However, many times we do not see it that way but we see it as something negative and painful, which we want to avoid, however, to learn it is inevitable to go through these stages to be able to finally overcome them, we can take advantage of or waste this opportunity to learn something about ourselves.

Limiting barriers and gaps when we want to achieve something, simply show that there is something we do not know and that we need to broaden our knowledge and skills allowing us to be bigger people with greater skills and knowledge.

Once this barrier is overcome, this gap, to achieve our objectives and achieve the desired goal we will finally be able to realize that to have achieved it we have crossed a series of obstacles which allowed us to be better people and to be bigger people, with higher skills, which ultimately made us more skilled people and have overcome all these barriers.

This is the importance of learning, of the declaration of ignorance and of our ability to learn through obstacles, without allowing negative mental models and limiting barriers to stop us.

Rather, on the contrary, that our mental models help and empower us to cross these barriers that do not allow us to achieve our desired goals.

7 JUGDGEMENTS

The judgments belong to the declarations. The declarations are different than Affirmations.

When we make a declaration, the words guide and the world happens to it.

They are like verdicts and with them we create a new reality, which only exists in language.

The judgments are an example of the generative capacity of language, that is, the capacity that through language we can create new realities.

The judgment lives in the person who formulates it.

People continually make judgments. When we communicate our opinions, we make judgments.

For example:

"Laura is an excellent communicator"

Judgments can be valid or invalid, depending on the person issuing the judgment.

Judgments are an important component of people's identity, and also the identity of companies, countries, etc.

When we see a person, we have many judgments. We are beings who constantly make judgments.

As people we have the ability to learn, so if before others considered (made the judgment) that we were:

"Bad at dancing", those judgments could be challenged by learning to dance or by mastering the dance.

When making judgments, we assume that as something happened in the past it could also happen in the future.

For example, the judgment "it is bad to dance", perhaps it meant that previously you had seen that person who danced very badly.

When we say,

-Juan arrived early for the meeting. (affirmation)

-It is very different from saying Juan is punctual (judgment)

In the second case, we are saying something that can or cannot be expected in the future, from this person or object.

There is something important also between judgments and actions. By changing our actions, we can change judgments about us.

Action generates being.

We act as we are. And we are how we act.

To the extent that we modify our actions, we can modify our being, and the judgments that are made about us, or that we make about ourselves.

The key to making a judgment is in the future, as we make judgments out of concern for the future.

For example:

"Samira does not know how to make reports", with this judgment we will prefer that someone else make the reports and not Samira.

When we say something, we reveal who we are. When we make judgments, they say more about ourselves than we say about others.

When we make judgment, we believe that we are only judging what we are talking about

But what we do not usually perceive is how much of ourselves we are revealing by making this judgment.

For example, when someone passes judgment:

"Juan dresses like a bum"

Not much is said about John, but about who makes that judgment.

If I say, for example:

"That city is gray and sad"

I will know something about the city, but more about who makes that judgment. (probably this person in this city feels sad and seems very gray)

Judgments always speak of those who make it.

EXERCISE

Mention some personal judgments

_____

_____

Delve into the judgments mentioned, and notice that these judgments say more about yourself than about the people you speak of.

8 BREAK OR BREAKDOWN

According to Rafael Echevarria in his book Ontology of Language "A break is an interruption in the transparent flow of life."

He mentions the following example:

"If while walking we stumble, we will suddenly see that pavement that was transparent to us before"

That is, what did not cause us problems before, now appears in our field of attention. From this event we seek to restore the "normal" order of things.

Every break involves a personal judgment of what happens. It is something that we did not expect to happen, and it is something that alters the expected course of things.

Every break is constituted as a judgment. (What for me is a break for another is not.)

-For example, we are calm doing a job on our personal computer and boom! the electricity goes out.

For some people this will represent a break, if we have to send our work for example.

But it might not represent a break for other people who live in our home.

And that's because they have different judgments than ours (they don't have the time limit that we do have to submit that work.)

This flow of things in a normal way is broken for me.

Every break is associated with a transformation of our judgments about what is possible.

There are negative and positive breaks.

For example, if the electricity goes out and I have to use electricity to work, it would represent a negative break. Since this would limit my possibilities.

But there are also positive breaks. If they call me, for example, saying that they have given me the job, it would interrupt my normal flow of things, and it would also be a break. My possibilities can now be expanded.

The break being a judgment is part of the person who issues it, and from this perspective we can indicate that the breaks do not occur "outside", but that many start from "inside" the person.

Since the break is a judgment, and a judgment a declaration, we can declare a break. Avoiding the necessity of waiting for things to happen.

For example, we can state "**I don't like my grades. I would like to improve them**".

This can be done in different areas of life, such as family, work, relationships, etc.

The declaration of break is important, first because it makes us aware of something that interrupts our normal flow of life.

Second, because **declaring breaks**, and given our competence and ability to solve and overcome problems, **can make our future and our world different,** since I am declaring and saying that is enough from a situation, **and also that I want to make a change or modification.**

EXERCISE

MENTION SOME NEGATIVE BREAKAGES IN YOUR LIFE THAT INFLUENCE YOUR LIFE (that disrupt the normal flow of your life)

_____
_____
_____
_____

_____

MENTION SOME POSITIVE BREAKS IN YOUR LIFE

_____
_____
_____
_____

_____

MAKE SOME BREAK DECLARATIONS THAT YOU CONSIDER IMPORTANT IN YOUR LIFE TO CONTINUE WITH WHAT YOU WOULD CONSIDER THE "NORMAL FLOW" OF YOUR LIFE

Example:

"I don't like the way my relationship is going. I would like to improve it. " (The fact that you do not like how your relationship is going, is a break, since it interrupts the "normal flow" of your life, the break is a judgment, and a judgment is a declaration)

_____
_____
_____
_____
_____

When we declare that something we do not like, or that it causes us annoyance, we can change it.

The breaks are judgments that tell us that there are things that we would like to change, and as through the declarations we can modify our world, also through the declaration of a break, we can establish the guidelines to change the world through of our words, this as we mentioned is a generative language.

9 THE COMPLAINT

Language generates action and if language generates action, what happens to the complaint?

The complaint brings out the negative side of things, it does not allow us to move forward and makes us circle around feelings of anguish and limitations, of resignation, of guilt.

This declaration influences our subconscious and does not allow us to advance as we are aware that language is generative, we are more aware and we are more careful with our words.

Knowing that the complaint generates new realities, but in a negative way, makes us more responsible when making our statements, since we know that our statements can also trigger emotions which directly affect us.

We all have dreams and goals and based on this we choose a job, a partner, we choose what to study, however, if we complain and only see the negative side of things, it will be very difficult to achieve what we want.

At all times we are making decisions and not making a decision is also a decision.

Choosing what we want to be is a choice.

We can also make the choice not to choose, but this is also a choice.

People are aware of this, and that is why we voluntarily choose the things we want to have in our lives, when this happens, the complaint disappears, since our language is positive and generative and takes us out of the role of victims or of feeling incapable of achieving something-

Believing that if we have the possibilities, that we are capable is a thought that give us power, and allows us to achieve the goals we want.

To achieve our goals, motivation and energy are important.

Positive statements give us motivation and energy that we will need to achieve our goals, if on the contrary we complain we will be taking away energy and taking power from ourselves, **or we complain or we start working on what bothers us, but not both at the same time.**

10 WORDS

Words are very important and you have to be very careful when using words. There are weak words that weaken us and there are strong words that empower us.

Words create our reality.

In coaching we say that language is not innocent, and after what has been explained above, I think you already have an idea of the importance of words and their power.

In fact, I once heard the following phrase: "the words of a person are the very expression of his soul."

In the bible it says: "and the word became flesh, and dwelt among us ..." (John 1:14)

One important character, for example, is the Japanese captain Yamamoto from World War II, who was the last to accept the war against the United States.

He was a person who did not speak unless he was to keep his word, he received death threats and was branded a coward, because he was one of the few who opposed the war with the United States, since he knew what it meant.

It implied that it was fighting with a nation, at least 10 times bigger than Japan, with a production that was four times that of Japan, with great resources and a great amount of human capital.

When he wanted to make a decision, he thought about it many times and was very aware that a person is his words.

One of my favorite characters is Napoleon who said the following phrase:

"The last to promise is the most faithful to deliver" Napoleon.

Those who promise the gold and the nose, but who ultimately do not fulfill anything they say, we consider them as charlatans.

However, those people who do what they say, we consider them people who deserve respect and appreciation.

Napoleon says this phrase, because when he asked his best generals for a very difficult task, they thought very well, and many times they rejected Napoleon's requests.

Napoleon, because he had goals to achieve, asked them to do it anyway, and asked them to keep their promises, those who took it more seriously, made calculations to see the possibility of achieving what Napoleon asked of them, therefore the last who promised to carry out these goals were usually the most faithful to meet them.

So, to be a more upright person, you have to do what you say.

I say it again, the last to promise is the most faithful to fulfill.

11 - ELEMENTS THAT DEFINE A PERSON

There are three powerful elements that define you as a person, those are:

- Your thoughts

- Your words

- Your actions

All three are very powerful and define who you are.

There are people who speak a lot but who do little.

Those people considered serious are those who speak and do what they say. These people are considered upright and serious.

12 - EMOTIONS THAT BLOCK LEARNING

ARROGANCE

In order to learn we need to open ourselves to the possibility that there is something to learn, an arrogant person is one who believes that he knows and does not need to learn something new.

Without a predisposition to learn, learning cannot occur, the harder the problem, the better our willingness to open ourselves to something new and question our beliefs, since it is so painful not being able and not having the ability to face those problems that eventually one goes on to say: "I admit, there is something that I don't know and that I am going to learn no matter what."

Success often generates security and security produces blindness. This blindness is usually associated with what we call arrogance, it is an emotion that tells us that we know everything that is known and that nothing and nobody can teach us something new.

When we are under the state of arrogance, we are not available for learning, for learning to take place we must have a state of predisposition to learn and of humility.

THE STATE OF RESIGNATION

This state takes away our power, we close ourselves to the possibility of learning, it closes possibilities for us.

What for others is possible for the resigned person is impossible, this person is not perceived as capable of achieving something specific, therefore his response to action is zero or very low.

That is why they say: "why am I going to do this? so that if in the end I'm not going to get any results".

This state does not allow us to move forward due to preconceptions that we have of ourselves, lack of confidence.

Phrases like: "why should I make an effort if they are not going to choose me?" Denote this state.

To achieve our goals, we need to have a predisposition to learn, a lot of energy and motivation to achieve the desired goals

We have to be aware of our emotional states in order to improve and exceed our goals.

THE STATE OF FEAR

Fear makes learning an obstacle, fear is usually linked to the experience of unworthiness, of lack of respect towards the learner, on the part of the one who holds authority in the learning process.

We are afraid of being mistreated, afraid that someone will teach us, show us our weaknesses, many times this happens in teacher-student learning.

Due to the fear of being judged the apprentice locks himself in a barrier of self-defense to avoid being humiliated, but he also avoids the learning experience.

Those who use fear or humiliation as learning tools are taking away the learner's confidence and preventing optimal learning.

Fear can also occur due to lack of self-confidence, fear, however, is also fought with education, when you educate about something you do not know, you reduce your fear of that thing that was previously unknown.

With proper education we can reduce the fear of anything or topic that we do not know.

HUMILITY

In the face of criticism, we are usually defensive, we resist criticism, we feel questioned as people in some cases we feel offended or ashamed and we blame external factors and dilute our responsibility, we justify unsatisfactory results.

However, it is easier to change ourselves than others.

Humility arises from improving what we can improve and not looking at others and blaming external things, but creating changes from ourselves in the things that we can change and influence.

By learning we expose ourselves.

When learning dance for example in front of other dance teachers and experts we expose ourselves to our ignorance, however, we must be aware that everyone starts this way and have the humility to understand that to learn anything we need to start from scratch and even if we are monsters and experts in other areas, because in others, we will be newbies.

Therefore, declaring our humility allows us to advance much faster since we will follow in the footsteps of that person who is an expert.

Many things that I have learned have been by people much younger than me in some cases, if I had taken an attitude of arrogance, I would simply have said phrases like "what is this child going to teach me?"

Humility allows us to learn from different perspectives from those people who learned and master certain areas, no one person can master all the science areas that humanity currently has, such as:

physics, chemistry, astronomy, finance, accounting, coaching and many more to discover, etc.

It would be very difficult for a person to be an expert in all these different areas that humanity currently possesses, which is why the declaration of humility is very important since many of these people who teach us are experts and have several years in these areas.

In some cases, they have dedicated a whole life to these areas so by using humility we can learn from these people, instead of questioning every word they say.

By declaring the state of humility, it allows us to be open to new transformations and new learnings, which will allow us to have a better vision that will help us in our lives.

13 - LEARNING MODALITIES

There are several ways of learning.

LEARNING BY IMITATION - Most of the learning that humans do is through imitation, we have a biological capacity to imitate that many species do not have.

We also have what are called **mirror neurons** that make us imitate what we see automatically, from the moment we are born we look at our world around us, the way others behave and we begin to imitate them, in this way we also acquire language.

When we see a baby laugh it is not because the baby has really laughed but because we smile at him and by mirror neurons the baby smiles back at us.

We tend to imitate what we see and behave how they behave around us.

Many times, we do not even realize what we do, we assume the patterns of our culture of our society and we do things without realizing it until many times it is internalized within us and we see it as something normal but this normality only belongs to a certain social system, when we change social system people could behave differently.

For example, if you travel to Japan, you will understand that the culture and its behavior patterns are different, for example, from those of Europe, which are also different from those of Latin America.

Only when we enter a different social system do we realize that what we thought normal, was not.

Learning by imitation is of great importance to our childhood and is maintained throughout the rest of our lives, it is determined by the past since we tend to imitate others, we learn more from what we see, than from what they tell us we should do.

MODELING

Once we notice the importance of this learning, we can talk about what modeling is, which is to take responsibility for the learning that we want to have generate in ourselves, under modeling we can imitate the behavior of certain individuals that we see as models.

Many of us have heroes like great soccer players, great tennis players, great businessman that we look up to and want to model.

Some experts mention that to be successful you have to model successful people.

If our authority in the social system that we find ourselves is high, then other people will begin to imitate our attitudes and model our behavior, this is how humans learn from each other.

LEARNING BY TEACHING

It is a process by which we learn knowledge and skills, this is observed in the educational system, what is taught in schools through videos, textbooks, what is taught in universities.

The social system predefines the learning content that the school will have, the social system defines what should be taught and mechanisms are established so that members undergo these learning processes. (homework,

exams, etc.)

Social systems can be very diverse, governments assume an important responsibility in guaranteeing that these processes are fulfilled, this learning system acquires a formal aspect and introduces elements such as hierarchy, authority and subordination, which constitute it.

Within these teaching systems, the student's ability to choose what he wants to study is limited, there are certain contents and topics that the system chooses as compulsory and that must be learned and passed at both a basic, medium and high level.

This system is also characterized by having certain doses of rigidity, a teacher-student relationship, the teacher instructs his student in what has been predefined that he must learn.

This learning is very different from imitation, it is a conversational process where it is sought that the student has the expected learning and the teacher is the agent responsible for ensuring said result.

Makes the teacher the main responsible for the result.

AUTONOMOUS LEARNING

I consider this to be increasingly important today.

It integrates the previous 2 as part of itself, it is an option for which we should prepare and that should be a priority task since under this learning we have the ability to choose what we want to learn voluntarily.

While in the teaching system it is oriented to dates and times and there is an order, under this autonomous learning **we can choose to learn what we want**, without having to wait so long or having to pass certain barriers, this way of learning is very important since it gives us the ability to learn by own will. The responsibility rests with oneself and leaves it up to the person himself to choose the learning.

The learner becomes the main agent of her own development and learning.

The person defines what it requires to learn and designs its own learning strategies, chooses the content of its learning, its sources, the times of the process and dissolves the obstacles that may get in the way.

He is responsible for the results of this process and has alternatives that allow him in some cases to combine types of learning.

He makes use of imitation learning in some cases, that is, he models other people who are successful in a certain area and does a form of benchmarking, to be able to do what the other person does and generate results similar to that person.

This learning also allows for introspection by comparing ourselves to other people and asking ourselves questions such as:

Why is he successful and not me?

Why does he make more money and not me?

What am I missing to achieve what this person is achieving?

We can also use learning by teaching, the person who learns has full availability to use all the tools that are within his possibilities to achieve the desired learning.

14 - LEARNING STYLES

People learn in different ways, each person develops their sensory capacities to different degrees, some people can be very auditory, others can be very visual and others can be very kinesthetic, that is, they learn more through the movement of their body.

Sometimes we think that we all learn in the same way and that we have the same abilities, but this is not usually the case.

VISUAL

Visual people tend to learn much more by observing, reading, many of them also have imaginative capacity so they can visualize different futures or alternatives, people oriented to learning in this way tend to see images, diagrams and reading material make use of photos, graphics, to illustrate ideas and points, they also have the ability to more easily remember when they have seen a picture or drawing

AUDITORY

These people learn better when they listen and speak, that is, they learn something more easily when they repeat them themselves or listen to something several times.

These people like to listen to audio tapes, they like to converse with other people, they like to discuss matters with friends and other people.

KINESTHETIC

These individuals learn through body movement.

This person learns through the use of his body, he likes to do practical exercises.

They prefer to learn by doing things, they like to write, dance, and everything that involves a movement of their body.

All people have the three types of learning styles, normally one of them is the one that stands out over the others in each person, however, we can have all three well developed.

For example, when we watch movies or series, we are using 2 styles that are auditory and visual, to learn many times we mix and use the three learning styles at the same time, to a lesser or greater degree all three are important.

-Identify which is the learning style that stands out the most in you.

_____

_____

- Identify the second and third most relevant.

_____

_____

Remember that all three are important when it comes to learning and when you want to learn something it is recommended that you use the three learning styles, the more channels and styles you use, the easier it will be for you to learn.

15 - OBSERVER TRANSFORMATION

For one person the food is delicious, for another it is a normal dish, and for another it is not delicious.

Why do people think differently in the same circumstance?

Good or bad, are subjective interpretations that part from the person who emits it, things are not good or bad, they are just things.

Each one believes that he perceives reality as it is, but in reality, each one perceives reality according to his perception.

So, what is the true reality?

There is no such thing since each person has a different way of interpreting reality.

For example, when you are a child the way you see the world is very different from when you are a teenager and the way you see the world as an adult is very different when you are a teenager.

So, we also perceive the world from a different perspective if we are men or women if we are tall or short and it also depends on the perception, we have of ourselves.

Faced with the same event, different people will have different ways of describing reality, it is as if each person saw the world from a different filter and this is because our life is based on:

-To our experiences

-to our belief system

-To our mental models

16 - MENTAL MODELS

¿ Is it bad to have mental models?

The answer is no.

What could be harmful would be if we consider that we have "the only" mental model or that our mental model is the correct one.

Mental models are part of a person and are present in the different areas of our life, on these perceptions that we have, we will make interpretations which will finally define our actions.

There are mental models that are positive and are called generative, that is, they respond to an attitude that we can change things, that we can create reality.

The observer that we are, leads us to certain actions, which ultimately lead to results.

We have to focus not on actions, but on the observer that we are, on our mental models, which ultimately leads us to interpretations of the world and defines the type of observer we are.

This observer will eventually lead us to specific actions that in turn will bring specific results.

The observer, on the other hand, is within a context, contexts such as trust, respect, understanding, allow the observer to work with greater freedom and these contexts are what allow the creation of new ideas.

Making each one a better observer will also allow us to design new actions that can lead to different or new results.

Mental models are images or stories that determine our way of interpreting the world and our way of acting, they can slow us down or they can also empower us.

These mental models arise from our senses in our perception of the external world.

Each person has their own mental models given our culture, our characteristics, physical, physiological, given our experience as parents, children, students, siblings and according to the roles we play in daily life, each one lives their own reality.

One act based on that perception according to that mental model under this modality we add to our mind aspects that we want or that interest us and we ignore others.

This is clearer when, for example, you want to buy or rent a place or an apartment for this you start looking around your neighborhood and you realize that there are several ads of this type and it is something that you had not noticed before because you never paid attention to it. (It was because we were ignoring them, and we ignore it because we are bombarded with information before which we have to filter the information.)

It is as if each person sees the world through a different filter, each person sees the world as they perceive it through her filters and not as it is.

This also has to do with our senses as humans, for example, a worm perceives the world very differently than a person.

A worm for example has limited vision and the way he perceives this world is very different.

A worm sees the world in 2d, its vision systems are very limited.

Humans have more senses, we perceive the world in 3d, but we are also limited by our senses.

Since according to Carl Sagan there is a bigger world, a world in 4d, or the so-called fourth dimension.

In this 4d world, due to our limited senses, we would be like the aforementioned worm, with limited senses and limited vision.

If you want to know in more detail what I explain, you can search on YouTube: "Carl Sagan and the fourth dimension."

Dogs, for example, can recognize more than 10,000 different types of scents, something that we cannot.

Therefore, we cannot say that we see the world completely as it is, due to the limitation of our senses.

We cannot see infrared rays, or radio waves, that are transmitted when we talk on a cell phone.

However, they do exist in the world, but as we are limited by our senses, we cannot see them.

The personal filters that we add to each person's perception ultimately determine the way we see the world.

There are limitations that make up our mind.

Richard Bandler and Grinder distinguish three limitations that are:

-neurological

-social

-individuals

Neurological Limitations

Neurological are tied to our five senses, one perceives the world according to the senses it possesses, under our senses it is how we represent the world.

Social Limitations

Also called socio-genetic factors, that is, categories or filters to which we belong as members of a system, given our languages, our customs, our roles in society, the perception we have about ourselves, the thoughts we have and the information. what we have just received.

A funny example of these limitations could be that the Japanese don't have the "L" word in their syllabary (they can't say "load", for example), and they can't hear it either.

The Chinese can't say the "R" word and they can't hear it either. (They cannot say "Rat", instead they say "lat")

If you laughed and you are a native English speaker, you may not distinguish the "b" from the "v", while the French can. (According to them there is a "huge" difference, I do not distinguish it either)

On the other hand, English speakers(and many other native speakers of other languages) cannot distinguish the 4 tones that Chinese language has, for example, they have 4 ways of saying "ma" in different tones and each tone means something different!

Individual limitations

Finally, there are the individual limitations, each one has a set of experiences, characteristics, personality traits and different temperaments, which help us to model a different world.

Our physiology also influences this way of seeing the world and the experience we live through our lives also shapes this perception of the world.

These differences mean that each person has a different way of thinking, a different mental model and different limiting barriers.

A fun example I remember is when I loaned a book that I read, to a couple of friends that talked about success, and it turns out that when I discussed the book with each one, they each focused on a different thing.

One talked to me about persistence to achieve success, he would mostly mention that part of the book.

The other person, on the other hand, touched more on the subject of a story mentioned in the book that had to do with age, the book mentioned that approximately people between 30 and 40 years old developed their maximum potential at this age, and that many people reached success at this age.

Which under his mental model had made a very big impression on him.

For my part, I had perceived the book differently in a different way and what had impacted me the most was about the different ways that people had to achieve success, none of them achieved it in the same way and for each person the definition of success it was something different.

I was surprised because many times we believe that, **just as we perceive the world, others also perceive it in the same way,** this is not necessarily the case, in fact, to think that other people look at the world under our same filters and our same perceptions it can lead us to error and confusion.

Another very important and very clear example is when I worked for a company and the management had clearly established in a few lines a goal for all the workforce, the management perfectly understood these goals in a particular way.

But when this goal came to the workers it had a completely different meaning, that is, they spoke of the same thing, the same goal, the same objective, the same text, but the way of interpreting it was very different, even though it was the same text.

What management finally did was communicate and explain in more depth the objective that was mentioned because it was recognized and understood that the way in which workers perceived this goal was very different from how management perceived it.

Although everyone thought were talking about the same thing, and having the same understanding, they weren't.

The management, as I mentioned, then had to clarify all this in more depth so that we could all understand the message that they really wanted to convey.

Each person observes the world in a different way and also when he acquires more tools and greater knowledge, the way he looks at the world changes.

One can see the world differently today, then it did 10 years ago due to new experiences, new knowledge and skills acquired through the years.

Another important exercise that is beneficial in this case is what I do when I watch a movie.

Every time I watch the same movie, I find some details that I had not seen before, and it also happens that when I talk with other people about the film, I realize that some saw some details that I had gone unnoticed, such as scenes where it is focused the camera in more detail.

Our moods powerfully influence the filter we have, and the perception we have about the world, if we are with a lot of energy, a positive attitude because we will feel at that moment that the goal is easier to achieve and that there are not many obstacles or that we can overcome them.

If, on the other hand, we feel despair and a feeling of incapacity then it will be very difficult to reach the goal since we consider it too far away.

The mental framework we have, the mental model we have and the limiting barriers we have are very important when it comes to achieving our goals, which can enhance our goals or, on the contrary, limit us powerfully.

Our mind can be our greatest tool to achieve success or a tool that can limit us to achieve it.

17- MOODS

Human beings, wherever they are, wherever they live, are always immersed in certain states of mind. There is no way we can avoid finding ourselves in one mood, and looking at life from outside of some kind of emotional state, whatever it may be.

A state of mind, consequently, defines a space of possible actions.

Maturana argues that emotions and moods are predispositions for action.

Athletes know this very well. Their moods determine their performance and they know that if they change them, they can change what they could achieve as well.

When we want to coordinate an action with another person, we must ask ourselves whether or not that person's state of mind is conducive to the projected action.

If we happen to be in good spirits, the future will look bright. If we are in a bad mood, the future will look dark.

Each state of mind brings with it a world of its own.

We can recognize three primary domains, the domains of the:

- Body

-Emotion

-and Language.

They maintain coherence relations with each other, and thanks to this the phenomena of one domain can be reconstructed in terms of the phenomena of either of the other two.

We can observe emotional phenomena and act on them, from the domains of the body and language, for example.

Moods can be influenced through the 3 domains of **the body, emotion and language.**

If you are depressed, for example. You can influence your mood by making use of the 3 domains.

What you can do is to inflate your chest, look straight ahead, and put a dominant pose, such as putting your shoulders in a victory position (mastery of the body), this will positively influence your mood.

You can also **influence through language (language mastery) by making declarations such as "I am strong, I know that I am going to get out of this, I know that I have the strength to overcome this problem"**, which corresponds to language mastery, but If I say this with a low and depressing voice, there will be no coherence between the domain of the emotion, and the body.

Given this, we also have to use the domain of emotion, repeating the previous words, if **we say these words with a strong tone and a good intonation and with a lot of energy, then we will be influencing our state of mind by making use of the 3 domains.**

To influence our moods, we have to influence at least 2 of the 3 domains.

A conversation is a combination of language and emotions.

Moods can be presented and reconstructed in linguistic terms.

We can influence our emotions through language.

And we can influence our language through our emotions.

18 - CONVERSATIONS

When there is a gap, a break is generated.

Very often we get "bogged down" in it.

As a way to examine this connection between breakdowns and action, it is important to explore the various types of conversations that can follow a breakdown.

Seeing our internal conversations will tell us if we are moving towards solutions and action, or if, on the contrary, we freeze and feel immobile.

The fact that the light goes out of our home is not a break just because the power goes out, it is a break, when through a statement and a judgment, it becomes a break, which interrupts the normal **flow of life**

EXERCISE

IDENTIFY SOME GAPS THAT GENERATED BREAKS IN YOUR LIFE

_____
_____
_____

Did some of them immobilize you or are you currently immobilized? What do you think this is due to and what can you do to change it?

___

1. Conversations of Personal Judgments

The first thing to notice is that this conversation is limited to prosecuting the break, but it does not yet move us to take charge of it.

Moreover, with this, instead of taking charge of the break, what we do is deepen its explanation, in its justification, in its psychologization. We are looking for responsible, guilty, and, not satisfied with finding them, we now proceed to make judgments against them.

Phrases like:

"These things always happen to me!", "I'm always unlucky in love!"

"I always come last!"

These conversations do not generate a change, a judgment is made on the situation, and we stay in the situation.

2. Conversations for the Coordination of Actions

This conversation leads us to act and allows us to overcome the breaks.

In the conversation for the coordination of actions, we generate future actions to take care of the existing break.

Its objective is to achieve a change, and intervene in the current state of things. When we enter into this type of conversation, we try to change what causes the break or to take charge of its consequences.

We are changing things from their current state and we are producing a turnaround in the normal course of events.

If we are successful, we can usually hope that the break is overcome.

What are the actions associated with the conversations for the coordination of actions?

The linguistic acts that allow new realities to emerge are : requests, offers, promises, and declarations.

One of the most effective ways to deal with breaks is to ask for help.

The consequences of not asking for help are, therefore, usually the prolongation of suffering, ineffectiveness, isolation.

This type of conversation has the power to change the state of things.

3. Conversations for possible Actions

When we do not know what actions to take to treat a break, we have the possibility to start another type of conversation.

We call this a "conversation for possible actions."

This conversation does not directly address the coordination of actions to face the breakdown in question, but rather is oriented towards the action of speculating new possible actions that take us beyond what we now know.

This is a conversation with the goal of expanding our possibilities.

Sometimes we do not know what actions to take when we have a break, before this we can use this type of conversation for possible actions.

This allows us a space to get ideas, and expand our possibilities.

4. Conversations for Possible Conversations

In some cases, we cannot hold conversations with someone, before this we can have this type of conversation.

Conversations can be held to create conversations in the future that lead us to coordination of actions or possible actions.

19 - THE LANGUAGE

Human beings are linguistic beings.

Language is born from the social interaction between human beings, it is a social phenomenon and not just something biological.

There is also a domain that we all share; they are a set of shared signs and symbols that allow us to understand each other.

We identify sounds and give them a particular meaning.

This consensual domain occurs in social interaction.

The French, the English, the Japanese belong to different language systems.

We are biological beings with biological capacity for language.

And we are social beings, where language is born from social interaction.

GENERATIVE LANGUAGE

The conception of language as descriptive is called the passive character, and the conception of language as generative as an active character

Now we have not just one but two ways of interpreting language.

On the one hand, the language has a descriptive and passive character (Affirmations).

On the other hand, language also has an active character, which generates reality (Declarations)

And as we said, declarations have the ability to shape our world.

20 - MOTIVATION

Important motivations in people to make changes, for example, that I have found through coaching processes are:

- the pain of not wanting to be the same

- the fear that something unwanted will happen again

- the frustration of overcoming something that bothers us,

among other feelings.

Which if used properly can empower the person to strengthen that area of his life.

Example of a coaching process:

What do you want to work on in today's coaching session? ...

What would you like to achieve in this session and this week?

What step can you take this week that will help you reach your goal?

What do you commit to do to achieve this goal?

In the coaching process, the motivation of the person is also important to achieve the changes that we want, before this we can ask the following questions:

How would you rate your motivation to achieve this goal from 1 to 10?

To which you might reply: "I'd give it a 6"

What do you need for this 6 to become at least 8?

After seeing your motivation, the next question could be: **what things would stop you from achieving what you want?**

Frequent answers are: fear, laziness, idleness, disorder, lack of discipline, lack of planification.

After the coaching process, what is done is a follow-up, to see how the coachee is doing with his goals.

MOTIVATION TO ACHIEVE OUR GOALS

The motivation to achieve our goals.

It happens many times that we have the goal or objective, we have the date, we have our options (See GROW model in section III), we have seen that it is achievable, that it is realistic (See SMART model in section III), and finally we have the goal as a declaration and a certain date.

But at the time of execution or when seeing the results of the work on our goals, it turns out that many times the desired goal is not achieved, **this is due on the one hand by motivation, and another important part may be due to mental programming.**

That is, if we do not have the necessary motivation to achieve our goals then, even if we have the most beautiful and perfect plan, we are not going to reach our goal.

Our motivation must be high to achieve changes in a coaching process.

For example, if we want to lose weight and we want to do it through running, going around the park, but nevertheless it is extremely cold, if our motivation is not so strong as to go out for a run and achieve our desired goal, then we will not want to go out because it's very cold.

On the other hand, if the motivation is strong despite the cold, despite the inconveniences, despite the problems, **we will achieve that desired goal because we have a strong motivation and we have strongly visualized the goal we want to achieve.**

I recommend that each goal and objective through these tools we always visualize them as the desired state, since this will motivate us very strongly.

Also, to increase motivation, you can do the technique of visualizing the 2 futures (mentioned in section III), since in this **way you will be able to visualize your dark future (if you do not exercise in this case), and your ideal future** (where you are in shape due to the added sacrifice of exercising versus being crammed in your bed), this could be enough to motivate you and get you on the ball.

Another important thing that I see that does not allow people to reach their goals, is the **subconscious internal patterns.**

Although we consciously say that we want to have money or that we want to have the perfect body, sometimes unconsciously we do not want it or we are afraid of it.

A person can say, for example, that he wants to achieve a better income or that he wants to achieve a more athletic body, but if inside him, he feels like an obese (that is, he has a vision of yourself as an obese person), he will hardly achieve that goal.

To achieve this goal, he would have to break this subconscious internal pattern.

To achieve goals, it is important to have a good image of ourselves, it is important that **we know and believe that we can achieve the goal we want, because if we do not believe it internally, we will not achieve it.**

To achieve our goals, we have to fight with the weak person that we have within ourselves and bring out the strong and virtuous person that we have within us, if this fails, everything else will fail.

This part is also the part of the execution, for that reason as I say when seeing all our goals and our objectives well done, **it is important to see the internal part of the people, their motivation and also the internal image that the person has of himself.**

If the person has a very weak or poor image of himself, in this case he has to enhance his personal image.

If the person has for example a mental image of being a person who does not deserve to be successful, or who does not deserve to have the ideal body, then he will hardly achieve this goal.

The way to overcome this barrier is through positive mental conditioning, through positive phrases and through motivation and a strong will.

I want to say clearly that there are no easy paths.

There is the way of effort, and a strong thought and mind to achieve our goals.

If we cannot reach this state, it will be difficult for us to reach our goals, our mental patterns are important when it comes to achieving goals and our motivation and will is important.

WHEN THE MOTIVATION IS NOT ENOUGH

Many times, it happens that we are very motivated one day, but the next day passes and, boom, our motivation is gone, we become unmotivated, our mood is not right and we feel demoralized.

In this case we have 2 alternatives that I recommend:

1 - Let me explain it to you with a story-

I once asked a person who was a very successful athlete the following:

How do you keep from giving up when things go wrong?

To which he replied:

When things go bad you don't give up, you just try harder. If I lose, I continue with my game until I can feel satisfied with myself, until I feel that today I did something good with my life.

Even if it is just a game, I am supposed to want to be good at this game and that if I become a better player, I will earn more money and I will do better in life, I will have a more economically peaceful life.

If I'm losing a lot, it means I'm not doing my best, even if it's a game.

I also asked the following question:

How do you do not to be demoralized and depressed, and keep going?

The key is that even if you are depressed and demoralized, you have to keep going.

Always stick with your goals, no matter how you feel. that's the trick.

As I mentioned the words are powerful, and these responses that he gave me were very powerful, denoting the kind of person this athlete was.

2- Another alternative

Another alternative that I recommend is having strong mental programming or reprogramming.

If you are not moving forward in life as you would like, it is very likely that many of your mental patterns are holding you back.

As we explain in the limiting beliefs, it is possible that you have many mental patterns and limiting beliefs that work against you and that are limiting you and not letting you move forward.

The solution:

-Go leaving these patterns and limiting beliefs through education.

I recommend watching many videos on personal development, listening to successful people, listening to things that motivate you, watching stories and biographies of great characters in history.

See current success stories, learn from successful people, model them.

Copy their success habits. Listen to audio tapes, videos, etc.

All of these elements will reprogram your mind.

Above all, listen to the words these successful people say. Usually, successful people use very positive and powerful words and phrases, you can learn a lot from these people.

How a person speaks is how he thinks, and how that person thinks is an expression of his soul.

Hear how successful people from different branches speak, hear how successful athletes speak, how successful entrepreneurs speak, among others.

EXERCISE

Read a video, audio, biography of a person (or more than one) that you consider successful and that you admire, and write down the powerful words and phrases that this successful character says

_____
_____
_____
_____

If you do the exercise, you will see how many of these people are successful, committed, **and make powerful declarations, and the world lives up to their words.**

This part of the reprogramming is very important, because in many coaching processes that I did personally, I felt that I was not moving forward and that I was not making significant changes, even though I was following all the steps in the coaching process. But i wasn't progressing as it should.

I needed to reprogram my mind, end limiting beliefs and put bad habits aside, have discipline and effort to achieve my goals.

21 - HOW TO END BAD HABITS

Let me tell you a personal story.

It turns out that I had a habit as a young man that, although it was not addictive, nor did I consider it harmful, this habit was already beginning to cause me some discomfort as the years went by, since I had more responsibilities.

This habit was to play video games a few hours a week.

Due to my time was limited and I had more and more responsibilities, these hours could be used in other things, such as doing work, studying, or reinforcing my skills.

So, I was beginning to see it as a bad habit.

Since this habit was ingrained in me (like every habit), every time I wanted to kick this habit, I would say things like:

"But I need to de-stress" "I am not a machine" "which is a few hours a week, if you work hard too, you deserve it"

How did I change this habit for another?

With a declaration:

My declaration was the following:

"I need to work on this specific goal, (I had an objective to achieve and it was urgent for me), **once this work is finished** (this work was going to take a few months, so any additional time in my favor would benefit me) **I will be able to play the hours I want, so until I reach this goal, I will not play for a single minute "**

The result?

As you already read in the declarations part, **declarations** are powerful, and **they have the power to make the world conform to our words (active power of language).**

Any declaration also implies a commitment from the person who says it, if the person who says it is a person with great integrity and commitment, it is most likely that the declaration will be fulfilled.

As I made the declaration that you read above, I had to fulfill it, since it was a commitment that I had made.

So, I started to quit this habit.

The first days, I had almost a need to return to my old habit, my mind repeated the phrases that I mentioned lines above "it's only a few minutes" "you deserve it" among others.

To which I responded by saying: "I made a declaration, and therefore I have a commitment."

And so, day after day, there was this mental struggle, those phrases in my mind saying "you deserve it" and me self-answering "I have a commitment".

Finally, after a few days those phrases of "it's only a few minutes" or "you deserve it" stopped resounding in my mind, as I was full of conviction and firmness with my words and my commitment.

These additional hours, I could use them to spend time with my family, and also to use that time to achieve the goal that it was going to take me a few months to achieve and that I had set for myself.

HOW TO ACHIEVE HABITS

The way to achieve habits is basically doing small tasks of what you want, but continuously.

For example, if you want to have a good body and exercise, you could start by exercising daily for 5 minutes.

It is little, but as you do it more continuously, it will get easier.

At the beginning there will be a resistance from your body and your old habits to prevent you from doing this activity, but if you do it continuously there will be no problem.

Due to the frequency of your activity, as in the case of exercise, it will no longer be a problem for you to exercise for five minutes, after having acquired this habit, you can gradually increase the time from 5 to 10 minutes and then from 10 to 15 minutes.

But what do we normally do?

Many people go to the gym, and on the first day instead of doing five or ten minutes of exercise they do three hours of exercise.

The result?

That their body hurts so hard and the experience is so painful that they spend 3-5 days recovering, and then they don't think about going back to the gym again, their bodies are exhausted and the experience was unpleasant.

Once their bodies have recomposed, they no longer want to go back to the gym because in their mind it is generated a bad experience, the appropriate way would have been for example to start with 5 to 10 minutes of daily exercise and gradually increase it every three days or every week.

This is the way to acquire healthy and desirable habits and gradually stop the habits that we do not want to have, we all have habits.

Having habits is something positive, since they help us save energy, they are things we are used to.

To change one habit for another, it is important as I said to start small.

If we want to quit a habit, but we do not know exactly what we are going to replace it with, what will happen is that sooner or later we will return to that bad habit because the universe does not like spaces.

There the phrase that says "If you want something new, you have to let go of the old."

So the first thing you can do to change an old habit that we do not like, would be to fill it with another activity that, if you want to have as a habit, and gradually change it.

ACTIVITY

Make a list of all the daily activities you do.

_____
_____
_____

-In it, list your main daily habits.

_____
_____
_____

-Mention those habits that you would stop having, and instead list those habits that you would like to have

_____
_____
_____
_____

In this way, you will be clear about your daily habits and activities versus the daily habits and activities that you would like to have to achieve your goals.

The most effective way to achieve your goals is that the activities that will guide you to achieve your goals become habits.

By making an activity a habit, it will help you enhance it. learn more about it, and strengthen it as a skill or talent of yours which you can strengthen for your benefit.

The way to have the desired habits is little by little.

That is, to introduce new habits to our schedule gradually starting with 5 or 10 minutes a day and gradually increasing as the days go by, the frequency and amount of time we dedicate to these new activities or desired habits.

Getting into a new habit at first is difficult, because the body likes to save energy. And creating a new habit takes a lot of energy and is something that our mind detests, so to acquire a new habit we must overcome our mind (our reptilian brain) with great will.

The best way to do it is with small doses of time at the beginning, so as not to generate a bad experience and gradually increase these habits.

We have habits that we want, and others that we do not.

The desired habits help us to strengthen ourselves as people and help us to develop our potentialities.

Through the evaluation of our habits, we can ask ourselves questions.

Do you feel comfortable with the habits you have?

If the answer is yes, the person is most likely comfortable with the habits they have.

On the other hand, if you are not comfortable with the habits you currently have and that some of your habits are harmful to you, the activity mentioned will be very helpful.

It is important to imagine doing this exercise as you see yourself under your habits and activities that you do daily.

Who are you with?

What opinions do you have about yourself?

Do you feel satisfied with yourself?

Looking at all areas:

-the physical area

-the family area

-the economic area

Do you feel comfortable with these habits and activities that you do daily?

Is there something you would like to improve or change?

What is your ideal state and your ideal habits that you would like to have in 5 years?

EXERCISE

Evaluate the activities and habits that you carry out in the different areas of your life (family, work, personal), do you feel comfortable with them? Is there something you would like to change?

_____
_____
_____
_____
_____

Doing this exercise can be very beneficial, since when you are not in your ideal state you feel anguish, you feel discomfort, you feel frustration and when on the other hand you imagine your ideal state, you imagine a strong, healthy, successful person.

And the pain that this mental image causes is very strong, we can take advantage of this pain to do the things that we must do, which, although at the beginning they will be heavy and difficult to apply because changing a habit is very difficult, later it will stop to be difficult and gradually we will improve.

Reaching the ideal habits that we want to have; in this way we will be achieving the future we want and we will reach the adequate potential that we want so much.

By doing the exercise and imagining, listening, feeling what happens in your life when you make those changes, when you achieve those goals, and have those desired habits.

All this visualization will help you powerfully to achieve the goals you want, which will be a powerful ally to achieve the goals and to face the obstacles that you will face to achieve the desired goals.

Human beings do change, when we were children, we had a different vision of life and we had much fewer tools than we have now.

As we grow, we acquire new skills and talents which help us survive under these circumstances.

Every day we have the opportunity to be a better person and a better version of ourselves, it is up to us to develop the potential we want.

It is also important to ask ourselves why we want these goals.

What is the rationale behind these goals?

This will also help us and give us motivation to achieve our goals.

Using this technique is deliberately using our mental potential and our mind in our favor, since it will allow us to imagine and achieve the desired future due to the mental image that we have created in our mind.

The mind is very powerful, I would say that the mind today does not fully understand even 10% of the potential of our mind, it is really so powerful and capable of achieving so many things, but many times we do not know how to use it in our favor.

Through coaching and the techniques that coaching possesses, we can reach our full potential.

It is important to take into account that to develop great potential we have to feed our mind with positive things, on the contrary, if we feed our mind with negative things, bad news, poor information, outdated information then the mind will not be able to reach its Maximum potential.

On the other hand, if we nurture them with positive things, for example:

-positive teaching material

-Books about what we want to promote

-seminaries, courses

-we interact with people in that field

-we acquire new skills and new competencies

We are empowering and guiding ourselves towards that goal.

Everything that we see, we perceive and that our mind captures externally is the material that it will use later to reach the desired potential.

The inputs that we give to our mind are important since this is the material with which we can produce results later.

Our mind is powerful but many times we do not orient it towards some objective, if we do not do this then our mind wanders and goes anywhere.

If we focus on a goal and focus all our strength towards that goal, then the mind will be concentrated and will be able to develop its full potential.

If we do not give our mind a specific goal to achieve, it can become paralyzed without knowing what to do, or it will lead us to any path since we are not taking a specific goal.

To achieve a goal, the ideal is to make a declaration in a positive way, give it a specific date and see the options we have to move towards that goal.

We also need to use visualization to imagine ourselves reaching the goal.

By doing this, we will start our entire brain in that direction and we will give way to unconscious energy to achieve our maximum potential.

22 - USE OF THE 3 DOMAINS

How to create and enhance our habits through the use of the three domains and how to achieve our desired goals and objectives through the use of the three domains.

Once we have our goal, we have to use all three domains to reach it.

For example:

My goal is to lose two kilograms in three weeks, the declaration that I can make to do it using these three domains.

"_____ (Name) I plan that from today in three weeks I will lose 2 kilograms of weight"

To this statement we include the 3 domains, which are:

- the emotion

-the word

-the body

When **saying that declaration (word)** I have to say it with a strong voice of encouragement, joy, strength, those words have to be **accompanied with that strength (emotion)** and the way my **body is positioned also has to be a position of strength**, with outstretched arms as if to indicate that I can do it **(body)**.

Can you imagine José de San Martín, giving the declaration of independence of Peru, with a depressing voice and with his shoulders slumped? No one would have believed him! or they would think, what's wrong?

These 3 domains are important when it comes to doing things, there must be congruence between the three.

For example, if a person says that he is a very sociable person, this should be seen in all 3 domains, through a voice full of confidence (emotion), using words that denote his attitude, and a non-verbal language of confidence and approach. through his body.

If we see inconsistencies in the person in one of these 3 domains, it would cause us suspicion and doubts.

If you want to achieve your goals, you have to have coherence and consistency under these three domains. Many times, we can achieve our goals only by using two of these three domains

Imagine a person speaking about motivation, with his arms down, gaze down, and a droopy tone.

Would you believe that that person will be able to motivate others? You might think that he needs to motivate himself first.

EMOTION

Our emotion is powerful and can help us achieve our goals.

For example, no one would hesitate to mention that a soccer team is more likely to win if they are motivated. The same is to achieve our goals.

If we have positive emotions like joy, optimism, under this optimism under this filter and this mental model we will believe that we are capable of achieving many of our goals.

Under this emotion our voice and our tone that we will speak will be much safer and people will notice and feel that if we are the people capable of achieving this goal.

Emotion is a powerful ally when it comes to wanting to achieve our goals.

WORDS AND THOUGHTS

We are the result of what we think, the words we say and the actions we take.

The tone in which we say the words strongly influences us.

If you see an authority figure, if this person uses strong words, but he says them with a weak or low tone, no one will pay attention to him.

If, for example, another person with a thick military-type voice and showing signs of dominance and leadership with his body uses strong words and tells us something, most likely we will listen to him.

Words and thoughts are powerful and define our life, it is through our words that we create our realities.

What we say can become our reality, that is why we must be careful with our words, especially if they are negative, since they can slow us down.

Phrases like saying "I don't think I will make it"

"I don't think I will reach my goal this month"

and similar, can work against us when it comes to reaching our goals.

On the contrary, if we say

"I know I am going to achieve it" and we say it firmly and our whole body is in a position of success will give us the necessary tools to achieve this desired goal.

THE BODY

The body is probably much more important than the previous two because previously, before creating language, humans communicated practically like monkeys, if you have seen a documentary about monkeys, you will see that most monkeys make small sounds like "Uh uh" "oh oh".

But their main communication tool is their non-verbal language through your body.

For example, an ape will touch his chest as if saying "I am the boss here", and if the other also feels like a boss he will make the same gesture and they will enter into a conflict.

If, on the other hand, the other monkey shows submissive body language it means that he accepts that the other monkey is the boss.

The domain of the body is the oldest that humans have, so we are able to understand and perceive the non-verbal language of other people.

If we see that people look down, we could think that a person is sad or unmotivated.

Remember that when you have the goal you finally have to make a declaration and apply these three domains.

To make the declaration and achieve your goal, your emotion must be powerful as this emotion will help you go through difficult times, when you have problems trying to reach the goal.

Your words and thoughts should be looked at carefully, since this if this is not done, it is very likely that your own words and thoughts will limit you.

EXERCISE

If you are down, or you see someone down, make him look straight ahead, and to put in a dominant position, in a successful posture, with his arms outstretched showing success and then have him say some powerful phrase ("like I am strong, and can get through this") accompanied by strong emotion and tone, you will see that at least partially his (or yours) emotion of this person is going to be affected.

To change our habits and achieve our goals we need energy, everything that helps us empower and gain more energy will finally help us achieve our goals

23 - COACHING AS AN ALARM CLOCK

Coaches are awakeners of people, they open new perspectives and possibilities to coachees (clients), they help them to get in touch with their minds and awaken in them personal growth, powerful growth.

Making use of the tools of coaching, it allows him to expand possibilities, the coach gives new tools, so that his coachee can achieve his goals more effectively, awakening requires the skills of the coach.

You cannot wake others, if you are asleep, the first thing the coach does is wake up and stay awake.

The coach as an alarm clock helps others to get out of the hole in which they are, limited due to lack of knowledge.

The coach, through his help, breaks down limiting barriers, old habits and transcends conflicts.

The awakening arises from the fact that we realize something that we did not know before, that allows us to explore new possibilities and helps us to enhance our learning and overcome obstacles.

24 - MASTERY WHEN ASKING

In a coaching process it is important to listen and ask the right questions, through listening we can inquire.

Through the questions we are able to obtain information, we can also test hypotheses.

Through questions we can many times make the coachee describe himself.

The coachee does this through his own words, by answering his own questions, for this we need to ask open questions, which give him the possibility of expanding on the subject further, while closed questions simply end when he answers yes or no.

Einstein said:

"If I had an hour to solve a problem and my life depended on the solution, I would spend the first 55 minutes determining the appropriate question, because once I knew the correct question, I could solve the problem in less than five minutes.

Asking the right question is very important to knowing the answer, and you have to take time to ask the right questions.

The mastery of asking is one of the skills that the coach must master.

SECTION III- COACHING TOOLS

In this section we will discuss many of the existing techniques in coaching.

Some come from life coaching, others from NLP coaching, and many others from ontological coaching, which as I mentioned is where I developed.

These tools can help us improve our productivity, achieve goals through powerful statements and objectives, reprogram our minds, and achieve greater personal development.

Some of the techniques I have adapted and / or made modifications and in some cases some, I have discovered or created my own models.

TOOL #1 – GROW MODEL

This model allows us, in the coaching process, to understand and solve any problem we have.

This is born from the fact that the coachee defines an objective or a goal and its starting point, developing a course of action to create concrete actions, to achieve their desired future and move towards the desired goal, it serves to achieve a goal, improve a performance, change a habit.

The model is divided as follows.

-Goal (Goal)

-Reality

-Options (Options)

-Will (Will)

GOAL

Here you start with the specific goal, that is, what you want to achieve.

For example, the question may be,

What would you like to achieve in our session?

What goal would you like to achieve?

REALITY

Reality is important to see if it is feasible to achieve the goal we want to achieve, and how much we are doing to achieve that goal, some questions could be:

What actions are you taking to achieve this goal?

Are you taking any related action to reach this goal?

How many times or how long a day do you do things to reach this goal?

Are you happy with that performance, what do you do to reach your goal?

Do you think that doing the activities and the time you dedicate to current activities will achieve your goals?

Is there congruence between what you want to achieve and what you do?

And confirm that it is realistic, because, for example, if you want to stop losing weight, but you only exercise once a week, you are very far from achieving this goal.

For which it would be necessary to make some changes

OPTIONS

What we seek is to see what options we have to achieve our desired goal, and it helps us to think about possible solutions to the problems and goals set.

Some option questions might be:

What can you do about that?

What other additional things could you do to reach your goal?

What current tools do you have to achieve the goal you want?

In reality it is also important to ask the time,

In how long would you like to achieve this goal?

WILL (WILL, COMMITMENT)

Here your preferred solution becomes concrete actions, for each of these possible actions you have to score from 1 to 10, to see your commitment to achieve the desired goal.

They should at least have an 8 in terms of your probability of doing them, since, if it is below 8, it is most likely that you will not do it and therefore if your coachee gives you a number less than 8 in terms of commitment, what you could do is rephrase the question or ask:

What do you need to get your commitment to reach an 8?

EXAMPLE OF THE GROW TECHNIQUE

Pedro is 29 years old and works in the commercial area for which he has to reach a specific quota of clients, currently he is having problems reaching his commercial goals at work.

Using the GROW goals (Goal, Reality, Options, Will) we will structure our questions.

GOAL

The coach: What would be the goal you want to achieve after everything you mentioned?

Pedro: Well, I would like to reach my commercial goals without having many problems.

REALITY

The coach: What actions are you taking to achieve these goals?

Pedro: Well, the truth is, I do my best to handle things, but there are some things that I don't usually do because I don't feel very comfortable.

The coach: Like which ones?

Pedro: It is difficult for me to start conversations with people I do not know, that is why most of the clients I have obtained have been through friends or acquaintances, but my list has ended, and it is increasingly difficult for me to get clients.

The Coach: Under this scenario are you likely to reach your business goal this month?

Pedro: As I mentioned to you, it is taking me more and more to reach my goal because I contacted almost my entire list of contacts.

OPTIONS

The coach: Regarding what you mentioned to me, how could you improve this (starting conversations with people you don't know), what other options apart from this do you envision to reach your goal?

Pedro: Well, I know people who are very good at starting conversations with strangers, maybe I could ask some of them for tips. Another thing you could do is read a book about making conversations with strangers.

Regarding the options, maybe you could:

- Exchange my contact list with other people in the commercial area who sell other products.

-Maybe I could ask my contacts for 5 additional numbers to contact them and offer my product.

WILL

The coach: How likely are you to do the things you mentioned to me and how much do you rate each one?

-Well, regarding the exchange of contact lists, I could do it with a couple of people I know, and I give it an 8.

- I can ask for another 5 additional contacts from my existing contacts, I could do it initially with my most trusted contacts, and gradually ask my other contacts, regarding the score I give it an 8.

The goal GROW, serves to establish a goal, see reality, our options and finally see the will to apply these objectives, for which motivation is very important.

TOOL #2 – SMART GOALS

It is very similar to the previous one, but these include tools such as specific time.

Without a goal it is difficult to get the client to concentrate, setting goals is important to achieve our potential, since without goals one cannot measure something.

How can you measure your performance if you don't put a date to it?

For example, you might want to lose weight, but without a specific date it could be in a month or in 20 years.

That is why the importance of time reflected in this SMART tool.

-SPECIFIC

-MEDIBLE

-REACHABLE

-REALISTIC

-WEATHER

SPECIFIC

We start with the first. **Specific.**

For example, when the coach asks:

What do you want to achieve? you have to check if the goal the coachee is saying is specific.

For example, the coachee says:

-I want to be better (it is very generic.)

It has to be more specific.

For example:

I want to exercise two hours a day.

-I want to lose three kgs. in 1 month.

They are more specific goals

MEASURABLE

As Peter Drucker says

"What is not measured cannot be improved"

To improve something, we need to make metric measurements, so the goal initially set must be measurable.

For example, "I want to lose weight"

Is it a measurable goal? the answer is no.

For example,

"I want to lose 3 kilos of weight" it **is measurable.**

Since you are giving a specific amount.

REALISTIC / RELEVANT

These depend on the person.

Is the goal wanted to achieve realistic for the person?

This varies from person to person, what may be achievable for one may not be for another.

So, in this case specifically you have to ask your coachee, and if it is achievable for this person to achieve what he wants.

In the case of losing weight.

The question could be:

Is it achievable for you to lose 3 kilos in 20 days?

Depending on the person he is, his habits, this goal will be achievable or not.

Is this goal you want to achieve realistic?

Is this goal you want to achieve relevant to you?

Well, if it is, the goal is well defined, if not, you have to adjust it

For example

"I want to lose 3 kilos in two weeks"

Is it specific? Yes

Is it measurable? Yes

is it achievable? Yes, depending on the person

is it realistic / relevant? If it is, the last metric which is time would be missing.

TIME

The goal should have a deadline, because you could lose the weight in two weeks or in 20 years.

The concept of haste and time is important when it comes to achieving goals.

When will you start your goal, your goal?

An example:

"I want to lose three kilos in two weeks from 15 ... of 20XX."

Now to make this goal more powerful we have to change the word I want or desire to "I am going to" or "I plan" which are more powerful.

Since "I want" is a very weak word and does not give much power, because everyone can say: "I want to go to Peru" "I want to go to Mars" "I want this, I want that."

To be more powerful this statement what we can say is:

-I am going to

-I plan/I am planning

Then the goal would end as follows

SAMPLE OF A SMART GOAL

-I plan to lose weight, 3 kg in 4 weeks from… of… of the 20XX.

or

-I am going to lose weight, 3 kg in 4 weeks from… of… of the 20XX.

Words are very important, words are very powerful, **and saying, "I plan" or "I'm going to" instead of "I want to" can make a big difference.**

Goals set in this way are SMART goals.

EXAMPLE OF THE SMART TECHNIQUE

Laura is 33 years old; she feels that in recent months she has gained a lot of weight, which is why she suggests losing weight.

The coach: What is the goal you want to work on Laura?

Laura: I would like to improve my physical appearance, so I would like to lose weight.

The coach: So today we will work with the Smart goal.

SMART - It means Specific, Measurable, Achievable, Realistic and defined with a Time. Please, define your goal.

Laura: Well then, I would like to lose weight.

The coach: How could you make this goal more specific?

Laura: mmm, well I would like to lose weight at least 3 kg.

The coach: Is this goal measurable?

Laura: I think so, since I mentioned that I would like to lose at least 3 kg.

The coach: Is this goal realistic?

Laura: Well, I think so, I know several friends who lost 3 to 4 kg.

The coach: How long would you like to reach this goal?

Laura: I would like to lose weight, at least 3 kg in 2 weeks.

The Coach: With all of the above, could you make a goal that is SMART?

Laura: mmm (thinks).

"I would like to lose weight (specific)

at least 3 kg (measurable)

in 1 month from the following week" (time)

"I would like to lose weight at least 3 kg in 1 month" (achievable and realistic)

Finally:

"I would like to lose weight, at least 3 kg in 1 month from the following week"

The coach: Very good. But let's use a more powerful word, instead of saying "I want", you could say "I am going to" or "I plan", and regarding the time, could you please mention a specific date.

Laura:

"I plan to lose weight, at least 3 kg from… of the month of…. From the year 20XX) "

The coach: Great, Laura, so from this goal, which you have proposed, we can go to work and follow up to see the progress of this goal.

Laura: Sure.

In this way, Laura was able to make her goal SMART, that is, to be specific, measurable, achievable, realistic and with a specific date.

TOOL #3 - ALTERNATIVE FUTURES

I have created this technique as a result of the use and application of coaching in coaching sessions.

This technique can arise several times in a coaching process, I call it the technique of the two futures or the technique of imagination.

Let me explain how this technique works.

This technique makes use of visualization (which is very powerful), and allows us to see two different alternatives, if we take two different paths.

This technique is very powerful, since many times we do not see the consequences of our actions, therefore when using this technique, we can see 2 different possibilities.

The 2 questions are as follows:

Given the current direction you are taking in your life, how do you imagine yourself in 5 years? (Imagine it) Are you comfortable with this future?

After having imagined it, if the person mentions that he does feel comfortable with that possible future, then this person may not need coaching since the current course is probably shaping the future that he desires.

On the contrary, if this person does not feel comfortable with the direction his life is taking, and how it would be in 5 years, we can ask the following question

How would you like to be 5 years?

Then the person will answer your things like:

That he would like to see himself earning more money, that he sees himself exercising more, that he sees himself meeting new people.

This technique is important because when showing the two alternatives:

-On the one hand, given the current direction he is taking, you are making him visualize a future in which he is not comfortable.

- on the other hand, an ideal future, in which you feel satisfied and fulfilled.

IMPORTANCE OF TECHNIQUE

This technique can help **motivate people to make the necessary effort to achieve certain situations** that would not be achieved if the coach did not make the person visualize these two alternatives.

Something important that I have to emphasize is that sometimes a coaching process can be good, however, the person sometimes does not present changes.

For a person to have changes, there must be an internal process of change, an important desire to want to change things, if this desire is not strong enough and the custom and old habits are deeply ingrained, it will be very difficult to achieve changes.

That is why I mention that you have to work a lot on the personal and mental part, this added to a powerful motivation to achieve the desired changes.

There are important studies of people who smoked cigarettes for more than 20 years, who had early cancer or cancer, and although they wanted to quit their addiction to cigarettes, they could not do so, even though it was harmful.

Imagine other people who want to change to other simpler habits and that their life does not depend on it!

This is important to highlight, since to achieve changes in a person's life it is necessary to have strong motivation to achieve it.

For example, if you are used to watching television, the motivation to stop watching has to be so strong, for you to do it.

For example, if you want to exercise or have a more beautiful and athletic body, you have to push yourself, and if the motivation to do it is not as strong as the pleasure of sitting in the armchair, then there will be no changes.

One way to strongly raise people's motivation is to make them see these two alternate futures that I mention, since, by making them visualize a future where they do not feel satisfied, it can motivate them.

Making the person imagine a future that he does not like could cause frustration in this person, on the other hand, **by making him visualize his ideal future, because you make the person dream that he can achieve it and also give him a strong motivation to achieve his goals.**

In this case, the pain caused by the effort he will make to achieve his goal will be much less painful, than the pain he would have if he does not get the things you want.

Also, reaching goals after the effort required will be very rewarding.

So, it is more likely that you are more prone to make more sacrifices **if you can envision this future.**

It is important for a person to be able to visualize themselves as they want, to have the necessary motivation to achieve their goals, this technique can be applied in your personal life and in many areas such as health, money, love.

This technique can also be modified, and instead of going to the future, we could apply it to the present.

Example:

Are you what you would have liked to be 5 years ago? Do you have what you would have liked to have 5 years ago?

_____
_____

Here you have most likely achieved some things that you wanted to achieve and others that you did not.

What things did you lack to achieve? What do you think you lacked, so that you have not reached some goals?

_____
_____
_____

This is a modification of this technique and helps us focus on the present.

Since we are the result of our past decisions.

Other variants could ask the question using 3, 5, or 10 years. Depending on the context and what you want to achieve in the coaching session (there are short, medium and long-term goals), some goals are more relevant than others for us, and some goals are subject to specific periods (for example, the college lasts 5 or 6 years.)

EXAMPLE OF APPLICATION OF THE TECHNIQUE:

Juan is 26 years old; he wants to do a coaching session because he does not feel satisfied with the path his life is taking, he does not feel well at work, he feels that in these years he has made little progress in his work area, and that the salary he earns is not enough and he would like to earn more money.

So here we apply the 2 futures technique, and we ask him.

The coach: Imagine that, in 5 years, you find yourself in the same situation as you are now, would you feel satisfied?

Juan's response: In no way, if that were the case, would I be frustrated, since I feel limited by my income, I would like to earn a little more money to be able to buy some things that I cannot buy now.

The coach: Now imagine how you would like you to be 5 years from now?

Well, I see myself making more money, and thanks to that, I can give myself some wishes that I cannot now give myself.

I see myself eating at good restaurants with my girlfriend more often, indulging in some personal wishes, and traveling more often.

The coach: What things would prevent you from having that desired future that you envisioned a moment ago in 5 years?

It would prevent me from achieving that desired future, if I stay in the same position that I currently hold.

This could also be because I did not have a work plan to be able to move up in my job.

It could also be due to the lack of organization and planning that I don't achieve these goals, I feel that for now I am a bit messy and disorganized.

The coach: How would you feel if this situation happened?

Well, I would feel frustrated, maybe sad, I would feel that my life is going nowhere, and I would feel that I would be missing many good things in life.

The coach: So what do you need to have the desired future that you mentioned in 5 years?

Well, as I mentioned, I need planning, a little more organization, more confidence in myself to achieve my goals, I need to become more professional, since, if I were to be fired, but if I am a good professional, I would find a job elsewhere, since a good professional always gets called.

I would need to try harder, work with this vision that you mentioned to me, of my desired future, perhaps improving my curriculum through learning new skills, through taking seminars or diplomas that can help me to climb in my professional career.

I think that doing all this that I mentioned to you if I would be able to achieve that goal, in 5 years, and perhaps in less time, if I focus on my goals.

This technique can be applied to other areas such as family, money, the professional area, among others.

It is good to make people see 2 alternate futures, so that they can see both futures, **and make an active decision in which of them they would like to create.**

You can apply this technique with yourself, and then apply it with other people in coaching sessions.

After this visualization, you could apply the SMART technique, to set goals and make a declaration.

This method helps us to see a clearer picture of the goals we want to achieve, the obstacles we would have, etc.

TOOL #4 – WHEEL OF LIFE

This is very important to see, all the areas of our life that we have and that we consider relevant.

We have areas such as family, work, personal development, financial goals, health.

You can add those additional ones that you would like to have, but with these we already have at least a specific framework.

Some important areas can be:

- the money area

-the health area

-the community area

-the family area

-the spiritual area

- the affective / couple area

-fun area

-friends

Usually, those areas that we find difficult to deal with or deal with are where we have the most problems.

EXAMPLE OF THE WHEEL OF LIFE

Fabricio is 27 years old, and he wants to see the wheel of his life, something that his coach had mentioned to him in previous sessions.

So, he and his coach begin to work on his wheel of life.

The coach asks Fabricio which are the areas that he considers the most important.

Fabricio mentions that they are:

-The family

- the love of a couple

- money

- health

- the professional area

- personal development

Then his coach asks him to score from 1 to 10, each area of his life, with 0 being the lowest and 10 being the highest.

Fabricio begins with his score:

-Family 8

- Love (of couple) 7

- money 4

- health 7

-Career 4

- Spirituality and personal development 6

Based on the above, we make Fabricio's wheel of life.

WHEEL OF LIFE OF FABRICIO

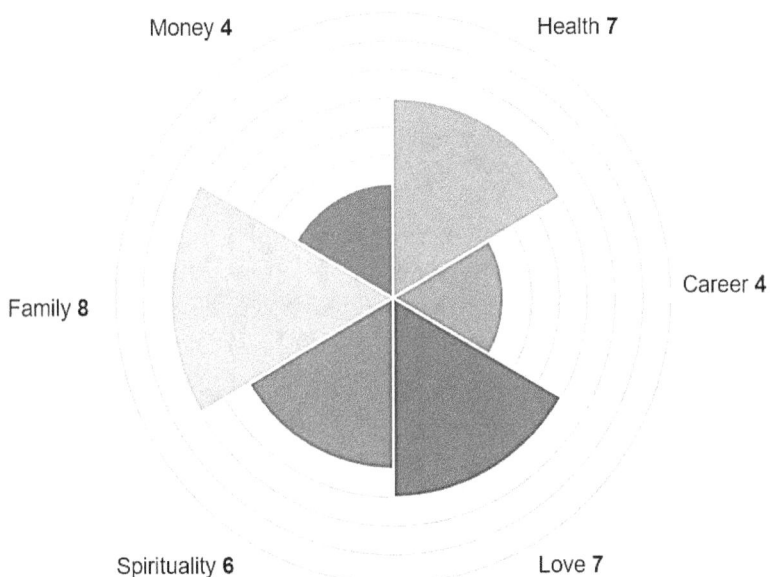

For a wheel to function optimally, it needs to be balanced.

We can see that Fabricio's wheel is relatively well in the area of health, love, family and spirituality (6+), in terms of money and career his wheel has a low score (4), which makes his wheel and his life have trouble turning.

Under these parameters, Fabricio could be recommended to promote these 2 areas of career and money, through a coaching process.

We usually avoid those areas in which we are worse.

The only way to face and overcome them is through awareness, and the humility to admit that we are failing in these areas so that we can work on them.

The good thing that the wheel of life shows us those areas that we have a low score and we must reinforce.

You can work on your own wheel of life, and remove some of these areas or increase others such as friendship, fun and others that you consider relevant.

Once the wheel of the person's life is made, we can continue with the SMART goal, and work on one of the areas in which they have the greatest weakness.

Finally, on the specific area (for example, money), we would set the SMART goal, with the aim of improving the score in this area until reaching a point where the person feels satisfied.

EXERCISE

Make your own wheel of life, and work on those areas that you need to improve, on these areas use SMART goals, to improve in these areas.

You can do it manually, or find on the internet, wheel of life simulators.

TOOL #5 - PROCESS GOALS VS RESULT GOALS

Not all goals can be controlled.

For example, you can control the goal of going for a run daily for 30 minutes, or reading a book for 2 hours.

But you cannot control the goal of "being hired", as it is determined by the company you are applying for.

You also cannot control the goal of getting "customer x" since that decision is not entirely up to you either.

But there are things that you can control, for example, in the case of looking to be hired, you could, for example, measure the number of jobs interviews you attend, the times you apply for a position through the different types of websites.

These would be process goals, which would be declared as follows:

"I am going to / I plan to apply for 10 job offers for the position of ..."

PROCESS GOALS

Process goals are completely under your control, and they are small steps that you take, to finally reach the result goal.

They are small processes that you carry out that will finally lead you to the goal of the result.

The process goals also have a detailed execution plan with various activities to be carried out to finally achieve the result goal.

Process goals are important since they focus us on the goal, looking at the immediate details that we must solve and do, they also allow us to avoid getting frustrated, since at least we are taking steps towards that goal, they also allow us to get feedback, to see how we are, regarding the outcome goal, and in some cases reformulating the goals (because after seeing the results, the goals could have been very optimistic or unrealistic)

It could happen that we want to lose 9 kgs in 3 months, for example.

So, the first month we should have lost 3 kgs, if we see that the first month, we only lost 2 kgs despite having done our best, we could reconsider the goal, and set it as losing 6 kgs in 3 months (2 kgs per month).

This would help us to stay motivated and anyway losing 6 kg of weight is better than not losing anything.

Another thing that could be done is to put more pressure on yourself to achieve your desired goal.

Process goals, then, allow us to rethink our objectives, be more realistic, or put more pressure on ourselves to achieve our goals.

EXAMPLE

In the case of the interview, they would be, for example:

- Apply for 5 jobs through the different job portals every day.
- Attend "x" number of interviews
- Prepare my resume and make it a seller

☐ Review my performance against applications and see what I can improve (how fast they see my resume and apply faster to appear among the first of the list.)

☐ Review my performance in job interviews and see where I'm failing

RESULT GOAL

☐ Get the right job according to my professional preparation and job competitiveness and according to my salary expectations.

The result goal is the end goal, it is what you hope to finally achieve.

In some cases, the outcome goal is difficult to define or, as we mentioned, it is not entirely up to us.

Outcome goals in some cases, can be difficult for the person to achieve, and cause frustration if we do not achieve them, such as

-Saving $ 100,000 per year

-Lose 20 kg in 3 months.

- Get a job in 2 months.

Therefore, it is good to constantly see the process goals (which are small steps that we take, to get closer to the result goal).

The process goals are a series of processes that will finally lead us to the result goal.

How do you eat an elephant? Asked my coaching teacher.

the answer? You eat it, bite by bite, tablespoon by tablespoon.

Well, it is the same for our goals, **how do you achieve such big and ambitious goals?**

Through small, continuous and staggered process goals that will finally lead us to the final result goal.

The outcome goals in some cases do not depend entirely on us, for which the process goals will help us to achieve them. (as in the case of being hired)

In other cases, the result goals do depend on us, however, to achieve them, it will be important to achieve the process goals, since each step of these process goals will finally lead us to the result goal. (As in the case of saving, if it depends on us, but this being a big goal, it must be continuously measured through processes, to avoid losing ourselves in the goal and follow it up.)

TOOL #6 - THE LEFT COLUMN

One way to improve the way we communicate and introspect our inner thoughts is through this powerful tool called the left column.

It was presented by psychologist Chris Argvris.

Under this technique, on the left side everything that the person thinks are put, and on the right side everything that he really says.

This left column has valuable information about us, our judgments and thoughts.

EJEMPLO DE LA COLUMNA IZQUIERDA

LEFT COLUMN Inner thoughts and feelings	REAL CONVERSATION
Marc is good at his job, but lately his productivity has dropped, and I want to know why	Juan: Hi, Marc. How are we doing with the commercial goals? We only have 2 weeks to close the month
The clients are very demanding, and the competition is also behind them, I hope to be able to close contracts with them	Marc: Well boss, I'm working with a couple of important clients with whom I hope to reach my commercial goal this month
You have to close those commercial contracts, central management is nervous due to low productivity this month, not to mention that we have less and less time.	Juan: I'm glad Marc, close these commercial deals as soon as possible, remember that we are measured monthly and that we have less time, close those contracts these days.
Although our proposals are good, the competition also created new discounts, which is why it is making it difficult for me to get these customers.	Marc: Sure boss, I am aware of it, and that is why I am behind these clients bringing them the best proposals
These discounts enabled this month should have made everyone reach their business goal, but there are hardly any changes from previous months	Juan: You can offer them the recent discounts that the head office has enabled to win customers.
Our company's discounts are similar to that of the competition, and our prices are similar. Getting	Marc: yes, don't worry, I am offering them the best proposals.

clients is now more a matter of empathy and good personal advice	
I expect a lot from you, as central management expects a lot from me. We are in the first weeks of the month, so I hope you follow what you say, otherwise I will have to take other measures.	Juan: Ok Marc. I expect a lot from you this month. I am sure you will achieve your goal; we will talk the following week to see your progress. Seize the day
I have to achieve these goals, I hate pression.	Marc: Sure boss.

Obviously, a person can only see their own left column.

The left column is important to see our judgments.

Phrases like these, use to appear in this left column:

"He is inept"

"He is not good for giving presentations"

"He is unpunctual"

"maths are hard"

They are judgments.

The first step is to process these opinions, and put a subject to these statements.

"He is inept" to → I think he is inept

"Maths are hard" to → I think that maths are hard

A second step is to focus on the speaking subject.

I think he is inept → I find it hard to believe that he is not an inept, and I don't like the way he works.

Maths is difficult→I have a hard time learning math

In this way I no longer define the topic in particular, but the relationship of the person with the topic in question.

Since for some people mathematics does not cause problems to learn, and for other people English is not very complicated.

Example:

-Math is difficult (raw)

Step One - I think math is difficult

Second Step - I have a hard time learning math and I have never really liked it.

Another example:

-Your presentation was bad (raw)

First Step - I think your presentation was bad

Step Two- I didn't like the way you did your presentation and it's not the way I do mine.

Seeing the left column is important to see the internal narrative of oneself, to dismantle false beliefs, about some issues, which being our opinions we consider them as facts.

Observations are descriptions of objective facts.

Judgments or opinions are subjective descriptions.

When we describe facts or observations we are talking about the world.

When we make judgments or opinions, we speak of ourselves.

The left column is full of judgments, which we confuse with facts.

Seeing our left column helps us see how our mental models operate.

The purpose of the left column is to raise our assumptions and misunderstandings whose understanding will make us see our own thoughts and judgments.

The left column is not about telling the truth, or betraying ourselves.

But to speak my truth with dignity, respecting my thoughts and emotions and respecting the other.

The adjustment variable is not the thing or the situation **but the observer that we are.**

The variable of change is oneself.

TOOL #7 - THE CIRCLE OF EXCELLENCE

This is a technique of Coaching with NLP.

This tool is very useful since it allows us to remember optimal internal states that allow us to obtain an effective performance.

It is one of the fundamental processes in NLP to help the person to manage their internal states in an intentional way.

.

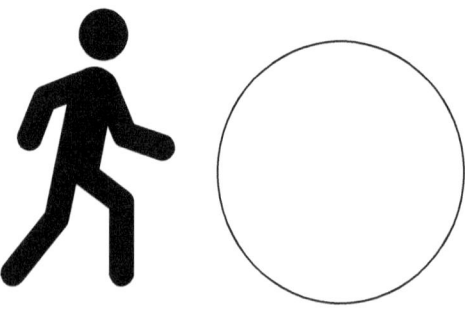

It allows the person to recover these optimal performances.

The steps are the following:

1- Draw a circle on the floor

2- enter the circle

3- Choose an internal state that you want to remember or that you need at the moment to face a challenge that you currently have. (like security, confidence, creativity)

4- Remember a moment when you had these qualities, close your eyes and remember it, remember the moment, the sensations and experiences (if what you want is confidence, remember a moment when you were full of confidence and security, feel it in your body you look at the posture you had when you were under that attitude)

Make it intense, while you do it, notice the cognitive and behavioral patterns that you had at that moment, both those that were evident and those that were subtle, in that state.

Look within.

how you feel? How is your face, how is your body? How are the sensations you feel?

Intensify this state and this quality that you had at that moment

5-Bring the present that attitude and ability, that behavior and that memory and feel how this can help you solve the obstacles you are having at this moment, feel it intensely once you have achieved it, open your eyes and get out of the circle.

By leaving the circle you can detach yourself from this state.

6- Try to re-enter the state you had when you were inside the circle and realize how easily you can enter and exit that state.

7-Repeat steps 1 to 6 until you get easy access to the desired state.

8- When you want to return to this state, to face some obstacles you can do it mentally and imagine a circle, you no longer have to draw it.

Doing this will help you when you want to overcome an obstacle by returning to an optimal state of mind that you had when you came to face a problem in the past.

TOOL #8 – PPEAR MODEL

"Insanity is doing the same thing over and over again, but expecting different results." Einstein

But it is what we often do unconsciously.

I created this model as a result of my observation of other models, such as the Osar Model that Rafael Echevarria presents in his book "The Observer and His World I", the model that T. Harv Eker presents called "Process of Manifestation" in his book "a millionaire mind", among others.

From these models I designed my own model.

Person (Inputs) → Thoughts → Emotions → Actions → Results

MODELO PTEAR

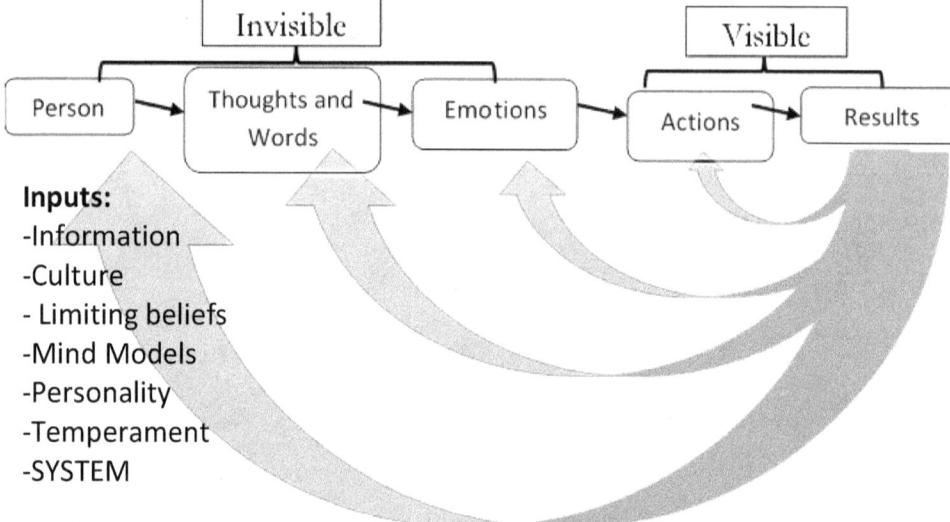

The person and his inputs:

A person is who is given his inputs:

-Their mental models, their limiting beliefs, their past, their culture, their temperament and their personality, their filters, their vision of the world, the information they have, the sources they turn to, in addition to this, the person is in different systems (you are a father, son, worker or employer, you have a nationality, a culture)

The systems as we mentioned can limit the capacity of action of the person, which can affect the changes that he can make. (If he is a worker, for example, his ability to act is limited according to the hierarchy he has within his company.)

Thoughts and Words:

We are the result of what we think. And what we think is based on our inputs that we mention (our culture, the information we put inside our mind, etc.)

They way we think, we transmit it through our words. That's why we say a person is its words.

Emotions:

Our thoughts lead us to have certain types of emotions.

Actions:

Our emotions lead us to take different types of actions.

Results:

Finally, our actions lead us to obtain different types of results.

The important thing about this model is that you can change your emotions if you take a step back, that is, if you change your emotions.

You can change your results by changing your actions.

But more importantly, you can skip the steps, going to the origin.

For example, you can change your results by changing your emotions.

And if we go more in depth, **you can change your results, if you change the person you are**, changing the inputs that can be changed and that also define a person (the person goes to other types of information, draws on new sources, break down their limiting barriers, etc.)

-**Some inputs can be changed** (such as the information we have, our mental models, our limiting beliefs.)

-**Other inputs cannot be changed,** because they are part of us, and are deeply rooted within us (culture, personality, temperament)

-And some can be partially changed, such as the systems to which we belong (we can change companies, but we cannot stop being parents, children, citizens, humans, etc.)

This tool, which I call the PTEAR model, helps us, since, if we are not achieving the desired results, we can go one step back in the model to achieve our objectives.

For example:

If we want to change our results, and we are doing it through our actions, but we do not see results, after using several and different types of attempts in this area, we can take a step back by changing our emotions, and we can even go back further, and change the person and its inputs.

Every time we make a change, it must be reflected in the results, we must constantly evaluate our results, and see in which area of the model we must make the necessary changes.

Something important to emphasize is that one of the most important variables that can limit our results are the systems to which we are subjected, since as I mentioned, the capacity we have to make changes in some cases to our systems is relatively limited.

. Visible Zones

Another important detail is that some areas are visible to other people, such as actions and results.

We see, for example, that the competition did this or that specific action.

Invisible Zones

On the other hand, there are the invisible zones.

These cannot be easily seen by other people or may be partially seen.

For example, it is difficult to know what the other thinks, the inputs that he possesses or the emotions that he possesses just by sight.

But these can be seen to some extent in some cases.

How can you see what is apparently invisible and make it visible?

-You can know what one thinks, listening to his words, as I mentioned a person in his words, his thoughts and his actions.

-We can see the emotions of a person through observing them, and if we have confidence with this person, we can ask how do you feel?

-We can know some inputs that a person has, seeing the characteristics of the person, seeing his culture, listening to the information he has, finding out what he reads, etc.

EXERCISE

What area do you consider that benefits you the most to obtain better results? Which one do you work on the most? In the end, is it the same to work on one area or another?

_____
_____
_____
_____
_____

Let's do a benchmark for: people and companies that we consider successful.

What things do they have that I don't? And what do I have that others do not? What do you think makes them successful? What things do you do that make you successful?

_____
_____
_____
_____
_____

In what areas are they different from you or your company? Are they in the visible or invisible areas? Describe

_____
_____
_____
_____
_____

TOOL #9 - ANCHOR TECHNIQUE

This technique is used in Coaching with NLP.

When you listen to a song from your "epoque" or some other song important to you, does it bring you any special memories?

If your answer is yes, then that song works as an anchor to trigger the experiences, emotions, memories or fantasies that you lived in that moment.

It seems that time goes back and you relive experiences as if it were happening at this moment.

But perhaps it is not only a song that makes you relive that experience, it may also be the aroma of a certain fragrance, some way of being touched, a place, seeing certain photographs, the taste of a dish, etc.

Anchors are visual, kinesthetic, auditory, olfactory and/or gustatory stimuli, which in themselves do not produce any physiological response in people, but which were associated with a particular physiological state to produce an internal response in the person.

It is important to consider the conditions to make or generate good anchors, these are:

• Make it intense and pure.

• Use unique stimuli.

• Handle it in the appropriate context.

As well as, take into account the types of anchors that exist, which are the following:

-visuals

-hearing

-kinesthetic

-olfatives

-gustatives

You can use this anchor, to recall a state of mind that you want to have to face a situation.

This anchor can be touching a part of your body, speaking with a particular differentiated tone, touching an object, making a particular pose.

When you use the anchor, you do it to anchor some state of mind, and when you want to remember it, you have to make that particular movement or sound to recover that state of mind.

EXAMPLE OF USING THE ANCHOR TECHNIQUE

Juan is an athlete, he had a very enthusiastic friend who lifted his spirits every time they lost a game, or every time he faced problems.

And every time he raised his spirits, he gave a little blow in his shoulder, his friend without realizing it, had created an anchor in Juan, every time his friend gave Juan a little blow on the shoulder, Juan responded with a smile, and was filled with courage.

Many years passed, and because they both went to study in different places, they stopped seeing each other.

Juan when he did a coaching course, they explained to him about the anchors, and he remembered this scene.

He realized that this blow to the shoulder was an anchor that he had, that could help him regain his spirits.

So, every time that Juan needed this state of mind to face obstacles, he would give himself a little blow on the shoulder, with the words and gestures that his old friend made him.

This comforted him and encouraged him to continue.

EXERCISE

Make your own anchor to recall the positive moods you need today.

_____
_____
_____
_____
_____

TOOL #10 - TECHNIQUES OF THE 15 OPTIONS

When you want to find solutions to something, and you need more ideas, I recommend this technique.

For example, you have the following problem:

-I want to improve productivity

So doing this technique you list 15 things you can do to improve productivity.

EXAMPLE:

15 THINGS TO IMPROVE PRODUCTIVITY

1- Work earlier

2- Seek more productivity through training

3- Raise the spirits of the staff

4- Take seminars to understand the psychology of people's behavior

5- Read a book about productivity

6- Give productivity workshops to workers

...

15- ...

And so, we are listing activities that we can do until activity number 15, when doing this exercise, you will realize that you can easily do it until the 5th or 8th activity, but from there it will not be so easy to have ideas to increase in this case the productivity.

This will require a little more concentration and focus, and in some cases, it will take us a little longer to come up with ideas to improve productivity.

It is important to take the time to list more possibilities, since many times, the latter can be very important solutions to solve the problem we have.

In this case, which is "improve productivity", the last 5 activities can be very important and some of them be relevant to improve the productivity of the person. You can apply it to improve your relationships, improve your sales, etc.

FINAL NOTES

If you got to this point, I want to thank you. I hope that the mentioned coaching tools help you improve productivity and get the best version of yourself.

I would be very grateful if you could leave me a review, to see what I can improve in later editions.

ABOUT THE AUTHOR

Max Chahua is a Peruvian coach and a CPA (Certified Public Accountant).

He has written books about Languages, Economics, productivity, finance, Coaching, and Accounting.

After working in the banking industry, and in the real estate industry, and finally in the accounting industry.

He began his career as a consultant, where he advises entrepreneur.

He also loves technology, has taken courses and seminars on digital marketing, has created applications available in the Play Store, such as "easy kana" to teach Japanese Hiragana and Katakana, and "learn Quechua", to teach the traditional Peruvian language.

He offers courses where he teaches digital marketing, auto-publishing on Amazon, and courses where he teaches how to sell their products or services automatically.

FINAL EXERCISE

I made some parts of my biography as a declaration.

Declarations are powerful, and have **generative capacity** (active language capacity), **declarations make the world conform to our words**.

For the declaration to also be fulfilled, the person who says them is important, if this person is committed, it is most likely that he will comply with his declarations.

Although I am an ontological coach and accountant, I put the writing of books in my biography as a declaration and therefore there is a commitment to fulfill them.

Before writing this book, I already had books written for learning languages (for learning Japanese), a couple of books about business, and the rest I will write due to commitment to my declaration.

This book completes one more step in the fulfillment of my declaration. (It's a coaching book)

I challenge you to write the biography of your life as a declaration, and use the active power of language, to model the life you want.

Make use of the power of active language, **so that the world adapts to your words through your DECLARATION.**

Write the biography of your life as a declaration, surely some parts of the biography that you would like to have, have already been achieved, and others you would like to achieve.

"Make use of the power of language and the tools of coaching to achieve the goals and objectives you want, and shape the life you want." Max Chahua

www.ingramcontent.com/pod-product-compliance
Lightning Source LLC
Chambersburg PA
CBHW072029230526
45466CB00020B/1149